W9-BZV-257

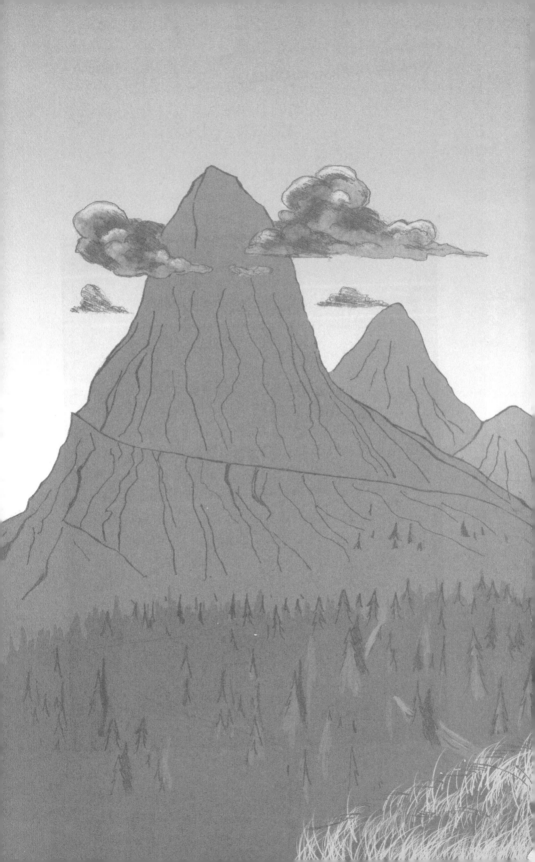

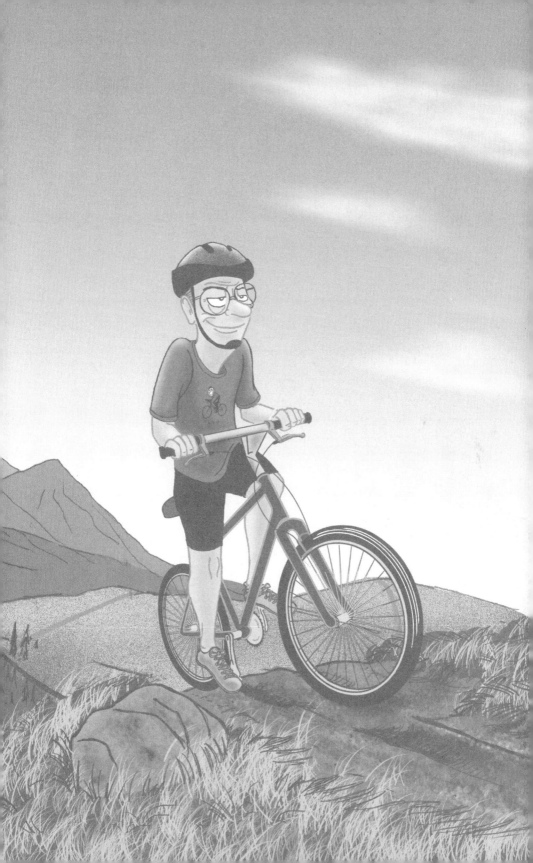

The
Ride Of Your Life

Fighting Cancer with Attitude

By John M. Ricco

with illustrations by Jeff Covieo

FERNE PRESS

Summary: A cancer survivor details the benefits of positive attitude both
in fighting cancer and in life in general. The main components needed to
achieve positive attitude are also explained.

Library of Congress Cataloging-in-Publication Data
Ricco, John M.
The Ride of Your Life: Fighting Cancer with Attitude /
John M. Ricco – First Edition
ISBN-13: 978-1-933916-22-4
1. Positivity 2. Attitude 3. Cancer survivors 4. Support groups 5. Mental
health 6. Oncology 7. Self-improvement
I. Ricco, John M. II. Title
Library of Congress Control Number: 2008920205

FERNE PRESS

Ferne Press is an imprint of Nelson Publishing & Marketing
366 Welch Road, Northville, MI 48167
www.nelsonpublishingandmarketing.com
(248) 735-0418

DEDICATION

For John L. Ricco, my father, who was a huge
motivator in my life,

Marian A. Ricco, my mother, who always,
always has a positive attitude,

Janice J. Ricco, my wife and bride of thirty-three
years, who was always there as
my caregiver; and throughout it all, continues to
be my main support,

my daughters, Christina, Carrie, and Cathy,
who have been and always will be an inspiration
for the joys of life,

and all the many individuals who were and
continue to be part of my support system:
relatives, friends, coworkers, and neighbors.

CONTENTS

INTRODUCTION

As a seven-year cancer survivor, I have felt the trauma of the cancer diagnosis. Through my own experience and talking with many other cancer survivors, it seemed that we all could benefit from a book to help us build our mental outlook through positive attitude, in order to help us as we go through the cancer journey. After all, why should each cancer survivor have to "reinvent the wheel" and not derive benefit from others who have gone down the road ahead of them? Why not share the knowledge and lessons learned? This book is meant to be a tool kit or "how to" for the journey through the cancer diagnosis, treatment, and life as a survivor. It reflects the lessons I learned going through the experience of cancer, as well as those of many other survivors I have talked to along the way. Additional insight was gained through discussion with doctors, nurses, caregivers, and others whose lives have been touched by cancer. This book will positively impact the lives of cancer survivors and those around them. It is a practical guide, based on real experiences and observations, to building a positive mental outlook that will carry you through the life ahead as a cancer survivor.

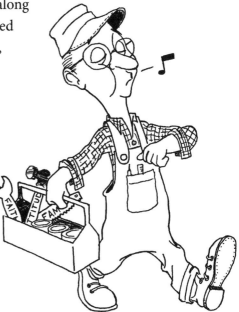

The key element to surviving cancer is a positive attitude. For me, it was what made the overwhelming difference. Despite the cancer "bump in the road," having a positive mindset for my life ahead provided me with the means to move forward. Additionally, I noted that others with a good attitude toward cancer and life also had an easier time coping with this disease. Attitude provides you with something bigger than cancer and helps you to get through the experience, move on as a survivor, and improve your life. Most importantly, it is the one thing you can control that can have a significant impact on your journey. Indeed, any major negative news or adversity that we as humans endure could be served by a positive attitude and the tools in this book.

My particular "flavor" of cancer was multiple myeloma, or cancer of the plasma cells in the blood and bone marrow. This is a blood cancer that accounts for only 1percent of all cancers. I was first diagnosed in June 2000, three days before my fifty-third birthday. The cancer was detected by the unusually high protein counts in my blood work from a routine physical exam in May 2000. At the time of diagnosis, I did not feel sick; in fact, I was feeling the strongest ever in my life due to extensive bike riding! Through the rest of 2000, I went through treatment, including chemotherapy, the high-dose chemo, total body irradiation, and finally a stem cell transplant in December. All the protocol got me to remission in January 2001.

In the chapters that follow, I have outlined some key drivers to a good attitude. Because I am a very active cyclist, I occasionally find good cycling analogies that help bring a point across. Fundamentally, dealing with cancer is like being on a bike ride. There are tougher parts (hills), and there are easier stretches (straightaways). Together, they are what life is all about: the ups and downs. The given is that the road is never totally flat and easy. We will be challenged and unexpected things will happen along the way. We must remain positive that we will get through this big series of hills called cancer.

As with anything worth doing, it is always helpful to know what the goal is. In this case, the objective is to get ourselves, as cancer patients, to the attainment of a positive attitude for our new path in life. It is early on in this journey through cancer that patients must sort out the view they will have toward the disease.

It is important to note that while I talk about a positive attitude in respect to the patient, this information should be used by others as well. Caregivers, family members, friends, co-workers, neighbors, and all others concerned with the survivor can benefit from building a better attitude. Not only that, but it will also greatly help for them to know what the cancer patient is dealing with mentally and emotionally. It serves as a basis for supporting those we love as they go through their battle with the disease. In other words, cancer is a learning experience for *everyone* involved.

Let's go down the road a bit and see what tools can help in the face of a challenge from cancer. We will see how certain basic approaches to cancer can make a big difference in the patient's outlook and how they feel about themselves while coping with cancer. Furthermore, a positive attitude will take you even beyond cancer and into the whole of life itself. It's an awesome ride!

> "You are today where your thoughts have brought you.
> You will be tomorrow where your thoughts take you."
> James Allen

Chapter 1
What is Attitude?

"My momma always said, 'Life was like a box of chocolates.
You never know what you're gonna get.'"
Forrest Gump

et's start from the beginning and talk about what attitude is. *Webster's Dictionary* defines attitude as "a mental position with regard to a fact or state." Notice that the focus is not on the fact or state (cancer, in our case), but on our mental position, or outlook, toward it.

Attitude, thus, is a state of mind. It is a conscious consideration of how we will approach our day. It represents a view of life, a way to approach day-to-day living. Of course, attitude can take many forms. We see this every day as we go about our lives. How do people look at life? This is the fundamental issue to consider when trying to define attitude.

Certainly our surroundings, past and present, have to affect our attitude. This might include a number of aspects, but family, religion, culture, and education probably impact our lives and our attitudes the most. All these experiences and exposures, good or bad, will reflect who we are and how we react as things come up in our lives. As we go through life, all our experiences will then tend to give us a particular predisposition toward new events in our life.

What also affects living is change. Change in our lives is something we all learn to expect. However, being told you have cancer is a change that is dramatic. As much as we learn to expect change, and as adept as we may be at dealing with it, we are rarely truly prepared for a change so dramatic. Our only coping tools at diagnosis are whatever mental and emotional experiences our lives have had up to that point. Cancer is such a new and traumatic experience that it requires big changes in our mental focus.

But what is really interesting about attitude is our ability to change it so easily, no matter where we have been or what we have experienced. It is important to note that all we require to change our attitude is a will to change it! This is what makes the possibility of a positive attitude an attainable state, which, in turn, will make living with cancer a much easier challenge. When you have a positive outlook on life, it is what makes life enjoyable and will open the door to making life easier.

Again, because it is a conscious effort, the choice is yours and in *your control*. If you have a choice, why not make it for the better? This is the most important thing to remember—*you control the choice!*

"Our attitude toward life determines life's attitude toward us."
Earl Nightingale, success expert

"A problem is a chance for you to do your best."
Duke Ellington, musician

CHAPTER 2
ATTITUDE: THE GOOD, THE BAD, AND THE UGLY

"Life is what we make it: always has been, always will be."
Grandma Moses

The chapter title might remind some of us (okay, at least some of the older ones of us) of the Clint Eastwood movie by the same name. It had the good guy, the desperados (the bad guys), and the ugly (really bad guys!). Our attitudes run the gamut in the same way as the characters in the movie.

As discussed earlier, our upbringing and environment play heavily into where our attitudes are today. We are what we are due in large part to how we were raised and the environment we were raised in. Our family, friends, schools, churches, and a whole host of other socioeconomic factors all affect our morals, values, and attitudes toward life. Given all the variables, it is no wonder that attitudes vary so widely from person to person. But suffice it to say, as a result of the developmental process, most of us have a decent attitude to begin with. We are reasonably contented people, or at the very least we are able to get through the ordinary ups and downs of everyday living. We do manage our lives decently.

However, there are those of us who just do not see things as positively as others. They are the ones who always seem to be grousing about things. Everything has a downside—the "glass is half empty" mentality. As a result, they tend to think of the worst and are not optimistic about their lives or what is ahead for them. Their lives are limited by the feeling that there is no upside to anything. The most "advanced" version of this attitude (the ugly type) is just downright depressing (sometimes quite literally) and not really fun to be around.

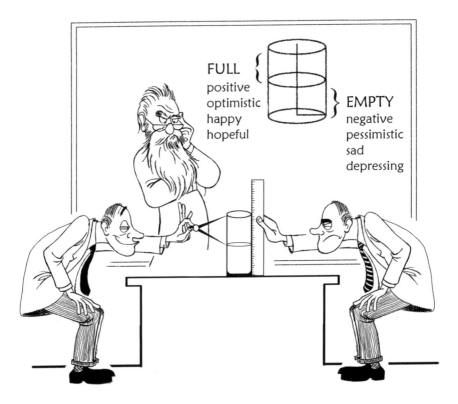

There are many views to life around us, but for our purposes it is enough to recognize simply whether they are "good" or "bad." We all develop some version of an attitude due to our given life experiences, and we live our lives in the context of that attitude. The result is that a person with a more positive outlook will have a more fruitful and enjoyable life. But life is full of changes and surprises. Now here comes the zinger—the doctor tells you that you have cancer.

We are never really prepared for a cancer diagnosis. We may be "conditioned" due to experiences with family or friends with cancer, but in no way can these experiences prepare us for our own cancer diagnosis. This is an initially traumatic revelation that hits hard. It completely changes our immediate view of the world, even for the most optimistic of us! There are the "why me" thoughts, the feelings of denial, the question of whether it could be a mistake, and the wondering what we did wrong to deserve this. Oh yes, then there is the question of "how long do I have to live?" It would be easy to become depressed and down on life.

Many of these negative thoughts come from the very frightening and deathly overtones that are associated with cancer. Cancer treatments, while much more "patient friendly" than even five or ten years ago, still can be very drawn out, take a pounding on your body and mind, and involve an abundance of tests, procedures, and treatments. Our emotional and mental strength are challenged many times over as we progress through the gauntlet of treatments.

When cancer hits, it has a profound and dramatic impact on your outlook toward life. When I was first diagnosed, I felt my whole life come to a screeching halt. I very much believed that the doctor made a mistake—the blood results were not mine; they really belonged to someone else. I could not understand why it was me with this diagnosis. I felt I was in really decent shape (okay, maybe five pounds overweight), and I had been doing a lot of biking in the previous five years. I was taking spinning classes (aerobic stationary cycling to music) three times a week, and as the weather warmed in the spring of 2000, I was doing weekend training rides of twenty to forty miles at a time. I generally ate pretty healthy and was fairly active in my lifestyle. When asked by the doctor how I felt, I said, "I've never felt better in my life," and thought that I probably was in just as good of shape as when I was in the army years earlier!

At diagnosis, in June 2000, all the projects and deadlines at work didn't seem so important. All my plans for doing the MS150 fundraiser bike ride in July went out the window because I would be in chemotherapy before the end of June. Everything in my life was on hold until I could understand what multiple myeloma was, how it was going to be treated, what the prognosis was for survival, and what this all would mean to my family. Literally overnight, my daily life of working, raising three daughters, traveling with my wife, saving for retirement—all of that changed dramatically. I needed a new focus and quick. How was my life ahead going to look for me and my family? How was I going to deal with all of this?

Every patient goes through a denial or shock phase after diagnosis. The length of the process of "acceptance" of cancer will definitely vary from patient to patient. It is a difficult time emotionally. Cancer totally changes your life and body. Though you may never be totally "happy" about receiving a cancer diagnosis, it is very important to work through the shock and denial to achieve an initial acceptance.

For me, it took about three weeks of mental deliberation to arrive at a point where I finally began to accept my disease. There were many emotional conversations with my wife and family during this time. My wife and I updated our estate planning documents. During that time, I had my first appointment with my oncologist/hematologist and had a round of chemotherapy. Around the third week, as the general treatment protocol and disease information became clearer, I came to the following point: "I have cancer, it is incurable, and I must deal with it. The good news is that there is a treatment process of chemotherapy followed by stem cell transplant, which has produced much greater and longer remissions."

You cannot wallow forever in the bad news that you have cancer. As difficult as it may be, you must get beyond the denial stage. Accept that you are sick and look forward, not backward, to your immediate future where the most advanced medical science will do its best to get you well. As soon as I was able to arrive in my mind at this point, I then focused on the treatment protocol, one step at a time.

Naturally, how advanced the cancer will be at prognosis will vary for every individual patient, and for some, the severity will be much greater than for others, but cancer never has to mean that you give up and don't fight it out. There are too many things that a person can do in their life to just say, "I'm sick, and it's all over." Of the many things that my parents taught me, one of the most important was my father's words when I was very young (which he repeated so many times over the years): "As you go through life and sometimes stumble and fall down; get up, dust yourself off, and keep going." In other words, DON'T GIVE UP! I have never forgotten those words, and they have been a very significant factor in my life. I feel it has been the basis that kept me focused during college, in my thirty-plus years in accounting and finance, and throughout my personal and family life. It has been a key part (if I may say so humbly) of my personal success. As I entered this new phase of my life, it became clear that the "fight must go on" and that I must get through this. I felt that acknowledging the disease and moving forward with a positive attitude was very important. I must be positive for my own health and mental welfare as well as for my surrounding family and support group.

No matter what sort of predisposition our upbringing and values instilled in us, we must reach a point where the answer is, "Let us beat this." Let us beat this so that we can get on with life and the things that are important to us and to our family and friends. You need to be as strong as possible with cancer, with a focus riveted on getting to remission and success. There is no question that your life is forever changed in that you have cancer, but being positive about the prospects is what will get you through it. I still have days when thoughts of mortality arise and bring tears. I don't think you really ever get over some of those emotions, but the spirit that drives us on is a positive attitude.

"What a man thinks of himself, that is what determines,
or rather indicates, his fate."
Henry David Thoreau, writer, philosopher

"It is not the mountain we conquer, but ourselves."
Edmund Hillary, explorer

Chapter 3
The Key Starting Point:
The Determined Fighter

"You play the hand you're dealt. I think the game's worthwhile."
Christopher Reeve, actor, activist

"Inside of a ring or out, ain't nothing wrong with going down.
It's staying down that's wrong."
Muhammed Ali, boxing champion

We must first identify one of the key tools for achieving a good attitude with cancer. The ultimate goal is a life that is more fulfilling and positive despite your illness. To do this you must develop what I call the "determined fighter" view. You must decide in your own mind to tackle cancer head on. Instead of moping or complaining about how dreadful this disease is, you must in fact be challenged by it to fight on in the face of adversity. Let it be the battle cry to arouse all your determination to "beat this." If you have faith in your doctors and medical staff to take care of their side of the process, then *you* must take care of your mind and attitude! You must consider this as one of those special challenges that can come our way in life. It must inspire us to be tough!

What we want to do as a determined fighter is to accept cancer as another of life's many challenges. It is another hill to climb on the road of life. No one says it will be easy, and you may undergo major changes to get through treatment. Despite the challenges to our body, mind, and emotions, we must feel we will prevail. We must believe that we have many things still to accomplish in our lives. There is so much out there awaiting us, and the world has needs in many areas. The determined fighter says (and believes) on a daily basis that cancer is not going to stop him from doing the things he likes to do. We believe we will get through this tough spot on the path. There is much to look forward to. Others will be inspired by our positive attitude that comes from being determined.

The determined fighter sees cancer as a gift. Yes, a gift! A cancer diagnosis is a chance to look at yourself in a renewed way. It is an opportunity for self-improvement toward a more fruitful life. It is a very clear reminder to do the best that you can on a daily basis. Cancer has been sent as a wake-up call for a positive purpose in your life. Survivors must take the view that we must be determined to live every day as much as we can. Cancer survivors can be one of the most motivated and energized groups of people, because they have the gift to realize the importance of life!

I worked in the business world for thirty years in various accounting and finance positions in public accounting and private industry. As the years went on, the managing of others consumed a greater part of my job responsibilities than the "doing" of technical functions from earlier in my career. It was fairly common to have an employee come in and state, "John, we have a problem." The employee was usually referring, of course, to some technical or procedural problem that just came up for the day. I would always shoot back, "Let's see if we can't make the problem become an opportunity!" We would then talk about the problem, and usually we could work out the situation so that some improvement—in business procedures, controls, customer service, profitability, etc.—would evolve out of the problem and make the business more successful. It seemed to take all the stress and the "woe is me" mentality and convert them into something helpful, creative, and positive.

Considering the "problem" (what an understatement!) of a cancer diagnosis, one must think of it as a positive instead of a negative. Cancer is not the end; it is the beginning of a new phase of your life. It is an opportunity to learn, grow, and realize something positive and new. In fact, this technique of creating positives out of negatives can apply to just about anything in your life, for that matter.

For me, I feel the positives took several forms. I believe I needed to slow down with my work and with my whole day-to-day lifestyle. I really did not "smell the roses" enough (even though I was an avid perennial and vegetable gardener—what a bad joke!). Cancer made me think a great deal about the things that are important in life and what my focus should be: family, friends, and the higher purpose my life should take. It has made me think more about the things that are all around us that we can easily overlook, especially some of the small things. At the risk of sounding sentimental, I really did start enjoying the birds singing, butterflies in the garden, blue skies, sunny days, and nature all around me.

I feel I am closer to my family. I do more things with my wife, and I talk more to the kids about things going on in our lives. Getting closer to my family has been one of the best results of my cancer.

It has also helped me to become more patient in my life. I am trying not to let things bother me that used to be so annoying and stressful before. Some of the most unimportant things, such as traffic, used to bother me immensely. More and more, I try to ignore these kinds of things. What is more important is that I am alive and in remission. It is time to make the most of every day!

It is certainly a time to count blessings. I have been blessed with a medical protocol that took me to remission. May it last forever! I have been blessed with a family, coworkers, and many other friends and neighbors who have supported me in every way possible. I have been given abilities and an education that have provided me with a long and successful career in accounting and business. I have been blessed to have parents who worked their behinds off to raise four boys, encouraged us, instilled sound values in us, and were always there to support us in everything we did. My father passed away from cancer some years ago, but he left a tremendous mark on our family's values with his wisdom. My mother is a very active eighty-year-old lady who has been and remains the ideal model of a very, very positive attitude. In the toughest of times, she was always steadfast in believing the best would come out of things. She always emphasizes the positive aspects of individuals and situations.

I feel cancer has inspired me to give back with some of my time. Having been blessed with a solid remission sent a statement to me that I cannot waste this gift. I must help others while I can. As a result, I am always willing to talk to other cancer patients and offer them encouragement. I have found that most patients love to share their experiences and help others with cancer. To that end, I have become very active with Gilda's Club Metro Detroit. Their multiple myeloma support group is certainly a great way for us all to pass on information, experiences, and hope for other cancer patients.

Additionally, I do volunteer work when I can as another way to help others. I get a steady flow of patient referrals from the Bone Marrow Transplant Link and the Blood and Marrow Transplant Information Network. I find great satisfaction in helping newer patients with their questions and concerns. As a member of my parish's Knights of Columbus council, I have been involved with many types of wonderful charitable service projects for my community as a whole.

When we become a part of these types of organizations, our lives become so much richer. I encourage you to seek opportunities to serve and help others in areas that are of interest to you. Giving of yourself helps others and, at the same time, provides you with another way to build a positive attitude. There is nothing bad to come from making a difference in others' lives.

In the journey through any adversity, it is important to have goals. Goals help you visualize what the target is and let you see where you are going. Cancer treatments are often a series of events. People sometimes say to me that my treatment phase must have seemed like a long time. While it did cover several months and was difficult physically, I felt it went fairly fast. The reason, upon reflection, is that if you look at each step in the treatment as the next goal, it isn't as daunting an experience. If you progress through each phase of the medical procedures with only

NEVER GIVE UP!

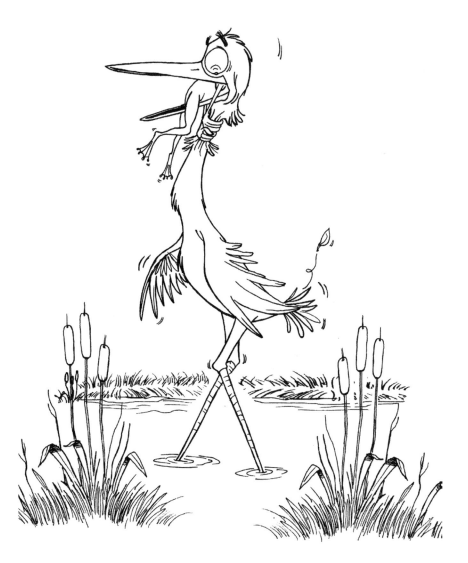

the next step as your goal, you reduce the process to smaller, easier steps instead of one large effort, and thereby it becomes less overwhelming. You also add positive feedback to your psyche, because you are sensing accomplishment along the way, rather than having to wait for the final treatment, which could be months ahead. In taking measured steps toward short-term goals, you will arrive at the overall goal.

We must make sure to be focused and determined to take our cancer diagnosis and turn it into a way to *improve* our lives and maximize our contributions to the world. We must be determined to fight through the negativity and make the most of the challenge to not let cancer get us down! Believe you can get through your challenge. You must have hope and find that there are many good things that come from cancer.

"If you're going through hell, keep going."
Winston Churchill, British prime minister

"The real glory is being knocked to your knees and then coming back."
Vince Lombardi, football coach

CHAPTER 4
THE PATH TO A
GOOD ATTITUDE: SUPPORT

"To know the road ahead, ask those coming back."
Chinese proverb

It is very important, especially in the early diagnosis and treatment phase, to build or find a support system. Support can come from many, many sources: a spouse, family, relatives, friends, church groups, coworkers, neighbors, cancer support groups (such as Gilda's Club), and others. Support also comes from internet resources, books, and magazines. It will quickly become apparent, as word spreads, that there are more people concerned about you and your success with treatment than you think. The support I received was incredible. I received calls, Mass cards, greeting cards, visits, offers of stem cells for the transplant, prayers, gifts, and more from a surprising number of people. All these things help to give you strength, determination, and a positive outlook.

I discovered through weeks and months of treatment that people are essentially good and very interested in the welfare of their fellow man. My faith in the human race, despite the daily negativity in the news, has been restored through the support given to me in so many ways. Before a diagnosis, when we are caught up in the daily rat race, it is easy to get frustrated and down on the real intentions of people. Road rage is a great example of this type of misplaced aggravation. After cancer, your whole perspective changes. What is important changes very quickly. Life is too precious! Family is more important! For many of us, the cancer diagnosis is a major change in our daily attitude and lifestyle.

If a member of your support group offers to help in any way, take them up on their offer! This is especially true if you are not able to move around as much due to chemotherapy or other physically draining aspects of treatment. You will need to conserve your energy for recovery. The treatment process itself can be stressful and fatiguing enough, so just let others cook your meals, get your groceries, or do whatever they offer. For many, this is not just a way of helping you, but also a way for them to cope with your cancer.

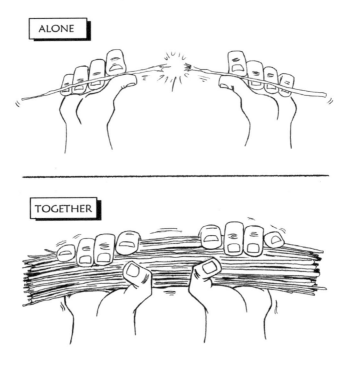

Knowing that people around you care is a great facilitator of a positive and optimistic outlook. Seek out a good caregiver who is willing to make time for doctor appointments, take you for treatment, be there for things needed to be done around the house, visit you in the hospital, and cover the innumerable details that come up. A committed caregiver is an essential building block for a positive attitude.

One tip that my wife and I learned during my treatment process was to keep family, friends, coworkers, and other support group members updated by use of emails. We created an update on a periodic basis, approximately monthly, to describe the current treatment and progress. Because so many people were interested in knowing what was going on, we found it much easier to put together a single email message rather than trying to update everyone through individual messages and phone calls. This saved considerable time, especially during the intensive parts of treatment where time was limited, and was effective in getting the word out to our support system. I highly recommend it to all cancer patients and their caregivers.

Another tip is to seek out organized patient support groups. Fortunately, there are many different support organizations out there, from those that provide general support and information to those that are focused on specific cancers. Some have extensive websites while others focus on face-to-face groups. There are many ways support can be presented, so seek out many different options and find the ones that suit you best. For example, Gilda's Club, which I have mentioned previously, has many organized activities and functions to support you, your family, and your caregiver. Gilda's has specific cancer support groups that meet regularly, and many other organized events, speakers, support groups, and therapeutic classes such as yoga, painting, and children's activities. They are one of many excellent support resources for cancer patients. In Appendix I, you will find information for many such resources—check them out for yourself!

One additional benefit from support groups is the social aspect. It is easy to become attached to the group and develop strong and lasting friendships, just like in any other place. I have personally met many great people in these groups, which has, in turn, provided many opportunities for social outings outside the group.

If group activities aren't your thing (and even if they aren't, I strongly suggest you give them a try), many cancer centers and hospitals have social workers and psychologists trained in helping patients through the cancer experience. They are usually available as part of a comprehensive service for cancer survivors and their families. Be sure to seek out these wonderful resources.

Speaking of great resources, the internet can be an immense source of support. Many sites will have information that can be mailed out to you, and others provide discussion boards where you can talk with other patients by leaving messages for others to read. These discussion boards are quite interesting and can be an easy way to ask a question or to read the questions and responses of other patients. The discussions can be as general as the nature of symptoms of the disease or as specific as what to expect with bone marrow biopsies, for example. Additionally, some sites provide chat rooms for you to converse online with someone who is familiar with your particular type of cancer. This is great for those who may not have an organized, face-to-face support group in their area. Refer to the resources and organizations listed in Appendix I, and try searching for others on your own. It is good to check as many sites as possible to find the best ones for you and your situation.

There are many great books that can be located at your local bookstore or library. Look in the self-improvement and inspiration sections, and don't be afraid to ask the librarian for ideas or assistance. I have listed several books for suggested reading in Appendix II.

As you can see, there are many sources and types of support available. Go to any and all areas for help! Do not be afraid to ask questions and seek out these information sources. Whether it is your doctor, nurse, a support group, peer support center, friend, neighbor, librarian, or whatever—learn as much as you can. Do not hold back from asking anyone. Seek out people and organizations to talk to, and you will be amazed at the support. As time goes on, you will be pleasantly surprised at how people will come to you to help in any way they can. All the information you gather will be helpful as a reference point or a way of cross-checking other information, and in the process you will gain confidence about what you are doing and where you are going. Doing this will build and bolster your positive attitude.

I believe it is important to do what you like to do and *do it now!* Get involved in activities, groups, organizations, specific interest clubs, hobbies, etc. Doing things you enjoy will bolster your mind and body with constructive and positive reinforcement. You will feel greater self-confidence and self-worth. Join clubs and organizations that will help you to meet new people who have the same interests as you. There is so much out in the world to do. Do as much as you can. We all have limits, due to physical and mental strengths, but again, do as much as you can to whatever level fits your situation. One of the lessons of cancer is that you should not put off doing things. If you want to call someone, do it now. If you really think you should meet a friend for lunch, do it now. Do now what the heart says you should be doing! Be determined to live a life doing the things that you enjoy and you will draw support from all your activities, both mentally and emotionally.

"The capacity to care gives life its deepest significance."
Pablo Casals, cellist and conductor

CHAPTER 5
YOUR PARTNER IN CANCER:
YOUR CAREGIVER

"One kind word can warm three winter months."
Japanese Proverb

"Too often we underestimate the power of a touch, a smile, a kind word,
a listening ear, an honest compliment, or the smallest act of caring, all of
which have the potential to turn a life around."
Leo F. Buscaglia, author

C ontinuing with our desire to reach the goal of a positive attitude, we must emphasize the key player in our support system:
the caregiver. A cancer patient cannot do it alone; a caregiver is
essential to the process. It is very important to come up with a designated
caregiver who will help you during your downtimes when you physically
need help getting to appointments and treatment. Additionally, caregivers usually will run errands, do tasks outside the home, and even help
with tasks in the home, such as housekeeping, when you are in a weaker
state due to treatment and cannot do these things yourself. This is even
more important during the toughest parts of treatment, such as during
heavy chemotherapy, major surgery, or a bone marrow transplant—even
the strongest among us will be unable to take care of every last thing on
our own during these times.

Not only is the caregiver a significant part of the physical support
system, but he or she can also help greatly with the psychological aspects
of cancer. A caregiver is usually a spouse, relative, or close friend who

will be willing to commit to the time when needed by the cancer patient. It probably isn't a bad idea to have a "backup" caregiver in case your usual one is not available when needed. I was fortunate to have a spouse who could fill this role and who could arrange her work schedule with her employer to get me to appointments and such whenever it was needed.

The caregiver is the person who will step forward and agree to help you. He or she is your partner in the cancer journey. Caregivers are the unsung heroes of cancer! They are there to encourage with their words. They help when they give feedback to the patient and can also provide humor along the way. Sometimes, just a word of encouragement to the survivor will boost their day. Caregivers help to give us a mental "pick me up" when we have down days due to treatment and thus are a huge part of the psychological and emotional needs of a cancer patient.

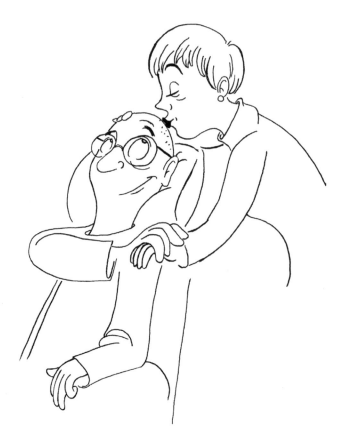

The caregiver, as your partner in cancer, also provides a very important role as a listener. Sometimes the cancer survivor needs someone just to listen when they need to talk about things on their mind. Some thoughts just need to be allowed to come out to help the patient heal or sort out things mentally. In some conversations, a caregiver can just listen rather than try to provide an answer or response to every concern the patient states. The patient in fact just needs to "unload" without expecting a response.

It should be noted that some cancer patients for different reasons do not really have someone close, like a family member or friend, who can act as the caregiver. In this case, another option is to view a support group as a caregiver. The group can act as a sounding board for the mental, emotional, and psychological needs of the patient. Additionally, someone in the group may be willing to help out with driving to doctor visits or even accompanying the survivor to tests, office visits, and the like. Often, you will find that two or three people will offer to share the caregiver duties if no single person is available to take the entire responsibility.

The use of humor by the caregiver in the daily process can be so helpful in easing the whole cancer experience. I have dedicated an entire chapter to this topic later in the book. Suffice it to say at this point that a little joking and kidding around, when done properly, will certainly make the caregiver assignment easier for everyone.

The caregiver is a key player in helping hold the family together and leading the support function in many respects. The caregiver, to me, is as much a part of the recovery and attitude process as the patient himself. There will be points along the way where you just can't do everything yourself. Your energy will be drained, and you will need the caregiver to step in. At other times, your mind may be weary and need a boost. Having your caregiver around at these times will truly be a blessing!

One of the most helpful abilities of the caregiver is that they can go with you to the various doctor and treatment appointments. At these appointments, the caregiver will pick up on tidbits of information regarding prognosis, treatment, and more that the patient may miss. As a patient, many things go through your mind during doctor visits, and it is hard to register everything that the practitioner will say. You can become preoccupied with the procedure or examination and miss key pieces of information. Or perhaps you are simply so tired that some things just don't register. Frequently, while driving home from an appointment, my wife would mention information that the doctor said that I really didn't hear or remember. It was very important to have both of us there so that we got everything.

Find a person who really wants to do the caregiver assignment. Many times a caregiver will step forward on their own because of their relationship with the patient. It is important for the caregiver to be comfortable with his or her role and be committed to the job! Note also that caregivers must take care of themselves—a sick caregiver is not a good caregiver. Allow some space and time for your caregiver to get a little "me" time along the way.

I really believe that a cancer patient cannot get through treatment without a caregiver. My wife says that I got to remission on my own and with flying colors. I told her that I couldn't have done it without her. A patient cannot do it alone. Sometimes it is the physical needs, but many times it is the encouragement with words or presence that gets you through all the chemotherapy, radiation, and multitude of tests and appointments.

To handle all the protocol, the general support system around you is critical. Their help and encouragement through all the emotional and psychological hardships are significant aspects of their role. The caregiver is the keystone to all the support, and is an equal partner in the care and process of treatment. The patient's mental attitude is greatly enhanced with the degree of support they receive from the caregiver.

> If there is a load you have to bear
> That you can't carry,
> I'm right up the road,
> I'll share your load,
> If you just call me.
> From "Lean on Me" by Bill Withers

Chapter 6
Keep Learning:
Information and Knowledge

"There is only one good, knowledge, and one evil, ignorance."
Socrates

"One who asks is a fool for five minutes,
but one who does not ask remains a fool forever."
Chinese proverb

Your support group will provide you with all the physical, emotional, and psychological support you will need, but you can also derive support from information. You must find as much information on your disease as you can. Even though I was diagnosed over seven years ago, I still bring a list of questions with me for each month's visit to the oncologist. In the early months, the list was a dozen questions or more, and in later months, the list has grown shorter.

A patient must *never* be reluctant to ask questions of any medical provider: hospital, cancer center, doctor, nurse, technician, or any other person treating you in the process. Sometimes medical personnel see so many patients that they can't possibly remember to tell you each thing. It is better to view the appointments and contacts with medical staff as a joint effort—they work to advise you of each new treatment or update, and your job is to ask questions in order to cover each step of the protocol as completely as possible. Knowledge is good for building a positive outlook. Understand as much as possible about your blood tests, chemotherapy, side effects, transplant options, radiation, medications, and anything else medically affected by treatment for cancer.

It is worth noting that your medical team of doctors, nurses, technicians, and medical centers is an extremely valuable source of information. They are your primary sources of knowledge. Ask questions whenever you meet with these people. There is always something new to learn or to review about your case. There are constant breakthroughs in cancer research and treatment.

Change, like the change in your health, must be monitored. Any information you acquire will only help build your strength in attitude to fight this illness. Lack of knowledge tends to build fear of the unknown. The unknown breeds doubt and sadness. So be a learner, and follow your medical team's instructions. If you frankly don't have confidence in your doctor, you should seek out another doctor in which you do have absolute confidence.

You should also listen to your body—this usually comes naturally to cancer patients as they are particularly sensitive to what is going on with their bodies. Discuss with your doctor any changes you notice. As suggested earlier, be sure to take your questions to the doctor with you each visit. Put concerns on paper so that they will not be forgotten. Do not leave the doctor appointment without getting answers to your questions. Any good doctor will respond to your questions. While doctors are busy people too, they will want to answer any questions that you have. Make sure they are aware at all times of all medications you're taking, any therapies being used, side effects of treatment, and any physical changes. Keep in mind that the "mental" side of treatment is as important as the physical side.

I cannot emphasize enough that you be your own advocate. By that, I mean that you must ask the questions that affect you. If you are unclear what the doctor or other medical professional has told you, you must keep asking until you are satisfied that you have all the information you need. Do not accept unclear answers; understand what your treatment is going to be. Get second opinions if needed. More importantly, know what side effects, benefits, and implications this all has to your specific situation. It is your body! Do not be shy about getting answers. Be determined in your fight to have the best for yourself as you move your life ahead.

Be sure to look for data and educational materials on your cancer everywhere you can. Cancer organizations have all kinds of booklets, tapes, and brochures on all the various aspects of cancer: treatment, medications, fatigue, pain, clinical trials, psychological issues, and the list goes on. Much of this material is free.

As I started the search for information early in diagnosis, I found the internet to be a wealth of knowledge. I have provided an extensive list of resources, including website information, in Appendix I. Check out any and all sites on cancer that you hear of, especially those specific to your type of cancer. There is a wide variety of information on most websites. Many of them also provide written material by mail, usually free, covering many aspects of cancer, and may even provide newsletters on a regular basis to keep you up to date. For example, myeloma has really good internet resources with the International Myeloma Foundation, Multiple Myeloma Research Foundation, McCarty Foundation, and others. Some of these organizations will gladly send good information on myeloma to you and even to family members as a way of getting the knowledge circulated.

You should also realize that clinical studies, new research, and statistics on your disease will be available as well. Sometimes these are fairly technical and can be quite frank in their discussion of things like mortality rates and responses to new treatments. Just remember to take that in the context of what it is, and always go back to your oncologist with questions about whether there is professional consensus about the findings of any given study or about how your specific situation relates to those findings.

Knowledge gives you an understanding and a certain level of confidence. With knowledge, you are at least reasonably informed about what is going on in your body. You will be more confident and positive about yourself knowing that you understand what you are dealing with on a medical basis. It allows you to have information that can be used in conversation with others, including your support group, to enable you to tell your story. This very activity of talking to others will ultimately build a positive attitude because it allows you to express yourself or get your feelings off your chest.

Another key to gaining knowledge is to talk with other patients recommended by your oncologist. The experience of other patients will be of great help in understanding what lies ahead as well as providing good knowledge from a patient's perspective about the treatment process and the disease itself. You will find that talking to other survivors is a tremendous source of information on the disease and prevailing treatments. While each patient's case may be somewhat different than the next, even within the same cancer type, there is always something to be learned that you had not thought to ask or your doctor hadn't thought to mention. You can gain contact with other patients from a doctor referral, by seeking them out in support groups, or even just by striking up conversations in waiting rooms or at a treatment center. Some of the most informative time I have spent was while I was sitting with a group of patients getting our regularly scheduled IVs!

Talking to other patients is very helpful in sharing your story, finding out how other patients are faring, and learning about different therapies.

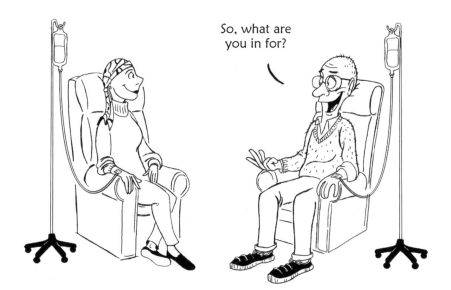

I have learned a lot about myeloma and cancer in general just by talking to other patients during day treatment or waiting in doctor offices. Ask your oncologist for the name of a patient or two that you could talk to early in your journey. I was able to do this with a couple of multiple myeloma patients recommended by my oncologist, and it was extremely helpful in understanding more about the cancer and providing first-hand information on the stem cell transplant process.

In addition to great disease information and support group resources, many cancer organizations sponsor family seminars and teleconferences that discuss recent treatment updates and countless other topics. Several even offer online chat sites, where you can send in questions about specific procedures and medications or express concerns about social or mental issues that have affected you. You can then see other patients' responses to your inquiries, and you can answer other patients' questions and concerns with your experience. Patients are one of the best sources for information on your disease, and these types of sites are great sources of support.

In a general way, when we study and learn new things, we add to our lives and to our positive attitude. Learning new things helps us feel worthwhile and more confident as we go forward. This impact from learning doesn't have to be just for the person dealing in adversity; it is good for everyone.

This concept of "keep learning" goes beyond just cancer. It is the interest in and process of continuing to learn about new ideas and the world around us. Sometimes our jobs or careers are the source of a need to learn more. At other times, it could be hobbies or sports that pique our interest to learn. In adversity, we have specific things related to the problem at hand that require us to investigate or become more informed. But beyond our problems, we can keep learning for the fun and enjoyment of it. By pursuing classes or learning on our own, we can enhance our knowledge level in our hobbies, pastimes, and other areas of our lives. In doing so, we expand our intellect, broaden our interests, round out our personality, and expand our understanding. Most importantly, we do something for ourselves that gives us a better outlook and a more positive attitude as we progress through life. We are uplifted and feel better, no matter what hard times we may suffer. All in all, if we keep an open mind and keep learning, we will feel better about ourselves and have a healthier attitude about everything. We will be more successful in the goal of living our lives fully.

As an example, over the years I have received great enjoyment from gardening—both vegetables and perennials. I spend time every winter studying how I can improve the beds for added color, blooms, height, and texture. As a result, each spring I have a few journal pages of changes to be made in the garden, which provide me with goals for this hobby. It creates a great activity for relaxing and clearing my mind of all the other "clutter and concerns." In addition, I have gained a tremendous sense of accomplishment and achievement from my hobby. I encourage you to keep learning. It is an opportunity to be something more for tomorrow than we were yesterday. This becomes an especially positive force in our outlook and our lives, particularly when dealing with adversity.

There are many, many resources for information out there. I have highlighted the most popular ones, but there are probably even more sources if you look for them. The main thing is to seek out any and all information to keep you up to date on all aspects of your disease and treatment. Be a seeker of information! Understanding all you can about your cancer and its treatment will help you in creating a positive attitude.

"Education is an ornament in prosperity and a refuge in adversity."
Aristotle, philosopher

"Nothing in life is to be feared; it is only to be understood.
Now is the time to understand more, so that we may fear less."
Marie Curie, physicist

CHAPTER 7
THE PATH TO A GOOD ATTITUDE: TALK ABOUT IT

"When life kicks you, let it kick you forward."
E. Stanley Jones

As part of the learning and information gathering process, it is essential to be as open as possible about your cancer, and to be willing to talk about it with others. Talking allows your mind to cope with your illness and, more importantly, to shape your attitude about it. By being open with family, friends, coworkers, and others you meet, you do two important things. First, you feel better mentally because you are not holding back and "hiding" your feelings. Being open and honest is less strenuous than having to dodge questions or skirt issues. Second, being comfortable talking about cancer allows others around you, especially the members of your support group, to gain strength from your willingness to be forthright about the disease.

It is important not to hold all your feelings about cancer inside. All the mental turmoil and agony of coping needs to be expressed, at least occasionally, rather than being bottled up inside. Those bottled-up thoughts will drain you mentally, physically, and emotionally. The stress alone is not good for cancer and your immune system. By talking openly about your diagnosis and cancer, it says to others that you have acknowledged you have cancer and are dealing with it the best you can.

It may be difficult at times to talk about it, particularly in the beginning, but you just have to start talking—once you overcome the initial

31

discomfort, every time you talk becomes easier. Eventually, it will be easy to bring it up frequently and let people know what you are trying to deal with and how it makes you feel.

When you discuss your cancer openly, others around you feel your comfort with the disease. Talking sends a signal to others about your attitude and your mental state. It allows them to understand, to some degree, the significance of cancer, both to loved ones and to society in general. If the survivor shows the strength to talk about it, those around them can also gather strength. It fuels a rallying of support for the survivor and in the process builds and enhances a positive attitude.

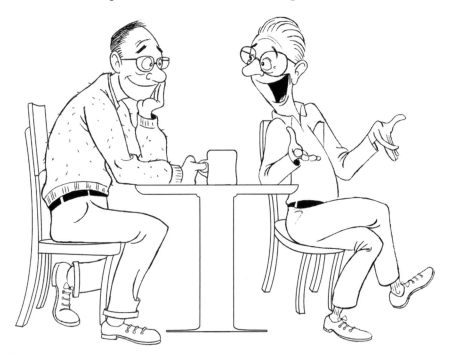

In many respects, talking about cancer also encourages others to talk to you. It opens up a dialogue for discussion and support. Seeing that you are talking about your cancer, others will feel more comfortable generating conversation. In this way you can then learn from them through the process. It is not a one-way street. By being open with others about your cancer, you will, for example, learn something from other people's experiences with cancer. In the process, you will gain more support and encouragement. When this happens, you are building your attitude in a positive way.

People around you, especially early in the process after diagnosis, will have a wide range of reactions to finding out about your cancer. Some will come up to you right away and give support. Others may hold back at first but will eventually come around to offer their support. There is also a segment of the population that actually is apprehensive and tends to shy away from approaching you altogether. They are undoubtedly afraid to approach you about what is generally considered a not-so-wonderful diagnosis! Being able to talk about your disease will help all of these people to be more comfortable about it themselves and will result in you having an even stronger support group.

People, in a way, are trying to understand the impact on you mentally, emotionally, and physically. For the most part, people want to learn what you are going through. They want to understand what the cancer experience is about, at least to the point of being able to help in some way. People want to help and show support. Talking gives them the capability to do this and facilitates acceptance of cancer.

I have told so many people about my cancer "trip" that it rolls off my tongue in daily conversation like talking about the weather! Inevitably, sitting in waiting rooms, in line at the post office, or at just about any meeting I go to, I end up telling someone my story. I am not saying that my trip with cancer is something special that has not been encountered by other patients. What I am saying is that talking about it greatly helps me to deal with the disease from a mental standpoint. It puts cancer out on the table, and I can put it into perspective as it relates to my life. Your personal story, as a cancer patient and as a survivor, helps explain who you are and where you have been. It also tells people that you accept (and can handle) your diagnosis, and, more importantly, that you are moving forward and looking to the future.

An easy way to get yourself talking about your cancer is to become involved with volunteer work, especially work that utilizes your experience with cancer. With this exposure, you can meet others who will be glad to exchange stories as you work together on the volunteer work. There are many organizations that need volunteers to do community service. Seek out organizations that match your interests, experiences, and desire to help. The bond that develops with this social contact and through your involvement can only bring about a positive feeling to you. Survivors are getting involved for a mutual good—it helps the patient, and it helps others in the community.

In general, we all look for real life stories that are optimistic. Hope is a contagious thing, and it is a great comfort to know that people can and do deal with cancer. When you tell your story, it will inspire those who hear it to do better in their own lives, knowing that someone with cancer has stood their ground and did not let negativism overwhelm them! It affirms that cancer has many success stories. It also says that cancer patients and survivors can do many positive things and have a great impact on the lives of others. Every day is an opportunity to do something good and to enjoy life. You do not have to be in perfect health to have a fruitful life. To the extent that cancer patients and survivors do this and talk to others about how good life is, then others around them will see the positive attitude and be inspired to look at things in a different light themselves. It should be in spite of illness or adversity that people strive even harder to have a productive and enjoyable life. A positive attitude is contagious!

> "The art of living lies less in eliminating our troubles
> than in growing with them."
> Bernard M. Baruch

CHAPTER 8
THE ROLE OF
RELIGION AND FAITH

"If God brings you to it, He will bring you through it."
Author unknown

I do not believe it is appropriate to force others on the subject of religion. It is a personal decision as to the role religion plays with cancer. It is up to each cancer patient to define or reach for any spiritual resources they believe in to help them through cancer. However, religion can be a great tool for building a positive attitude. Religion, or whatever beliefs in a higher authority you have, can greatly nurture you, sustain you, and help guide you through cancer. Religion points out that we need to appreciate the world around us and count our many blessings every day.

Religion and the belief in God or some other higher authority can have a very strong effect in pulling you through cancer. It can give you hope and faith that there is a bigger plan or reason for your cancer diagnosis. Naturally, each of us must define for ourselves what role religion will play in our lives. We come from different backgrounds and spiritual teachings. It is important that you address your spiritual needs in the way that best suits your beliefs. For me, a strong belief in God and a bigger plan is evident. I do not believe I am being punished or penalized with cancer for something I did wrong in my life. Although I am not perfect, I have always tried to live a good life. To me, cancer is a message from God to make a change in my life—to focus on doing more good things in life. It has become a wake-up call to spend more time with my wife and family and to give back to the cancer community in whatever way I can. Remember that there is always positive in anything that first appears as a "problem."

Faith is a very important part of the story of positive attitude. It is life-sustaining and, combined with prayer, is a huge factor for many, many people to get through adversity. Religion can carry us through the toughest of times. The teachings of God and our churches provide universal truths and all-encompassing guidance in our journey through adversity and life in general. We are provided with the power of God's love. It is a "plan" for daily living for all times. With faith, we believe that God is watching us always and will provide the path. Sometimes we need to pay attention on a daily basis for His signals or spiritual guidance. It is there, and we only need to be diligent about how we live our lives and interact with people around us. Others in faith will also provide strength and support in our journey.

One of the greatest realizations I came to was that being diagnosed with cancer was a gift. It may sound strange to those unaccustomed to the idea, but it is true. For me, it was a remarkable discovery. God wants us to understand that while cancer is not good for the body, it does bring us something good. The inherent good that cancer brings is a golden opportunity to change our lives for the better. Cancer can be a renewal of spirit and purpose and a wonderful chance to change and refocus our lives. We have been sent a sign to look at what is important for our lives and to compare how we have lived with how we want to live. What a great gift! This combination of faith in God and the opportunity that a cancer diagnosis brings to us is very powerful.

To understand that our faith and cancer will move us in a beneficial direction is huge. We must acknowledge God's impact, and then use the realization to proceed with our lives in a much more positive fashion. Our faith and refocus will provide us with a positive attitude for our lives. We will be energized to know that we have this gift to do more and better things with the rest of our lives. God is part of our support system! He is there to help.

With our faith and connection with religion comes a tremendous resource in the larger religious community. The most powerful support is the communal belief in God and the power of prayer. When we have many people praying for our trip with cancer, for our health, and for our well-being, we have many voices talking to God about us. It can be said that our support system has grown again! For those who believe, the power of prayer is great. It provides many voices and intentions for our sake as survivors. We are never alone in our journey with cancer.

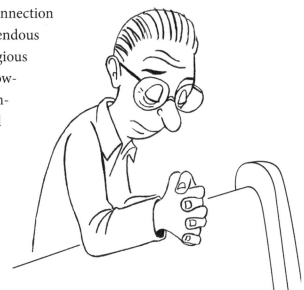

Cancer provides an opportunity to redefine your life and determine what is important. God is providing this opening to reassess what you should be doing with your life. How can you improve your life? How can you be a better person and do good things? What do you now define as the meaning and purpose of your life? These are all very basic, fundamental concepts, but sometimes it takes cancer and faith to force us to consider the options before us. Prayer and talking to God will send us answers and give us what we need in our adventure with cancer. Take time to assess this opportunity, and don't let it go away! Your life will have new meaning and purpose because of it.

During my cancer experience, I had a spiritual awakening. Working my way through the impact of diagnosis and months of treatment provided me with time for considerable introspection. I greatly reflected on the role of religion and faith in my life as it relates to my cancer. It became obvious to me that what was being pointed out by God was the meaning and definition of life. God was trying to help me move through cancer. The message was that I must be grateful for all my blessings. I have been very fortunate in my life in education, good parents, a great wife, three beautiful daughters, a great career in accounting, and the list goes on. Additionally and fortunately, I have been blessed with six years of remission with a cancer that has a five-year survival rate of just 32 percent. Reflection on these big items in my life, plus the appreciation for the little things, gave me guidance to the path ahead.

Change isn't easy, but each of us must begin somewhere and learn to move forward. I learned that I needed to slow down from the work rat race, enjoy my family more, and work on relationships with others. It also became clear that giving back and volunteering were where the rest of my life should be headed. My new purpose was to help others and somehow make a difference. This, for me, took several forms: volunteering with Gilda's Club and the Knights of Columbus council at my parish, doing peer patient support for other multiple myeloma survivors, and even writing this book. Not only does cancer refocus your life, but it can open doors to new things that you may never have envisioned.

I believe God is expecting us to do what my father always said: "Don't give up." You as a human on earth have a role to fill—a job to do—and you must do your best with what you have to make the world a better place in whatever way you can. I truly believe God has a plan for all of us, and sometimes, the signal to change comes in strange ways. I had so many prayers from individuals, families, and the church that I feel it certainly had a major role in getting me to remission.

Furthermore, it became apparent to me that God wants us to live our lives to the fullest and to maximize our contribution each day. We need to do this to the best of our individual abilities. We all have feelings, interests, talents, love, and aptitudes to share. Each of us is unique, and we all need to contribute to a better world. Individually and together and with God's help, we can make a real and significant difference.

Learn to appreciate both the big and the small; do not take things for granted! Religious belief is bigger than any adversity on earth. It is an eternal life aspect that goes beyond illness and challenges. If you have not experienced religious belief yet, I encourage you to consider it. For many people, it is an essential part of their resources to develop a positive and forward thinking attitude, not to mention adding strength and meaning to their lives. Religion and faith can sustain you above all adversity.

When I am down and, oh my soul, so weary
When troubles come and my heart burdened be
Then I am still and wait here in the silence
Until you come and sit awhile with me.

You raise me up, so I can stand on mountains
You raise me up, to walk on stormy seas
I am strong, when I am on your shoulders
You raise me up, to more than I can be.

From "You Raise Me Up" by Brendan Graham

CHAPTER 9
MORTALITY AND COURAGE

"Brood about death, and you hasten your demise. Think positively and masterfully with confidence and faith, and life becomes more secure, more fraught with action, richer in achievement and experience."
Eddie Rickenbacker, aviator

"To have courage for whatever comes in life—everything lies in that."
Mother Teresa, missionary

MORTALITY

Religion and the hereafter bring us naturally to the topic of our own mortality as human beings. There is no escaping that cancer brings mortality up close and personal. The topic comes up virtually immediately with a cancer diagnosis. Cancer forces the consideration of the possibility of one's own death from the realm of the purely hypothetical to the realm of the startlingly real. Thoughts of mortality will challenge our positive attitude, but the tools in this book provide us with ammunition for the fight.

The urgency or ability to procrastinate is not easy when you have a cancer diagnosis. Contemplating our own mortality is one of the most difficult subjects we have to handle as cancer patients. Thinking about death is about as fun as playing with a rattlesnake! It is not a subject people generally seek out for contemplation! But it is the fundamental "whammy" that affects someone with cancer. The biggest reason for this is the negative image that cancer has in our society. Perhaps "negative image" is being too tactful! People are scared to death (pardon the pun) about having cancer! There is so much of a negative stigma associated with cancer that patients will have it weigh heavy on their minds. Others around them will drop their mouths when they find out that someone they know has just been diagnosed with the disease. Great emotion and negativity tend to come packaged with cancer.

The widespread nature of cancer in our society certainly isn't a secret. The incidence rate of cancer is very high in the United States. According to the American Cancer Society's *Cancer Facts and Figures 2007*, there are approximately 10.5 million people living with cancer in the U.S. today. Additionally, the American Cancer Society reports that in 2007 there will be an estimated 1.4 million people diagnosed with cancer, and about 565,000 people will die of cancer. Cancer is the second highest cause of death after heart disease. If you consider the impact a cancer diagnosis has on immediate family, there are literally tens of millions of people in our country that are impacted directly by cancer. These are staggering numbers; unquestionably cancer has a major impact on health care in our country. It affects so many lives that it is very difficult to avoid it. This disease is so widespread that there are very few families that are not affected or do not know of someone who has had the disease or is currently dealing with it. With the prevalence of cancer, it is very difficult for a patient to avoid being affected to some degree by the dark side of this illness.

Furthermore, there are few cancers that have a *cure* from a medical standpoint, and most people are aware of this. Almost everyone knows of someone who has had to deal with cancer treatments, and knows what a toll treatment can take on a person. Treatments can be stressful, long, and sometimes dangerous. However, this is not to say that treatment protocol, medications, and procedures have not improved!

Research has made great strides in the development of new approaches to therapy. Much of the improvements have come in recent years, but great amounts of research continue every day. In fact, even more "patient friendly" treatments are available and continue to progress. Visit just about any cancer website, and there are all kinds of clinical studies underway for all types of cancer. Great progress in cancer research is being conducted and many exciting therapies are in the pipeline and on the horizon. Remissions are improving and getting longer. Also, the newest research and information on the human genome holds additional possibilities for understanding new treatments for cancer, exploring the links between cancer and DNA, and understanding the causes of cancer, in order to ultimately help find a cure.

In my disease, multiple myeloma, the number of options with new protocol and medications has grown very significantly in recent years. The options available for myeloma patients are much greater now than when I was diagnosed in 2000. The key is that the rate of development and improvement in treatment is occurring at an ever-increasing pace. I am greatly encouraged by all these changes. Many other types of cancer are experiencing even greater progress.

The main issue is that the public in general is keenly aware of the aggressive nature of cancer and the impact of treatment on the patient's physical health and mental state of mind, but is not very knowledgeable about the great cancer-fighting advances of modern medicine. There is great hope to be had, but let's face it—even cancer survivors go through significant weight changes, hair loss, change in coloring, and significant lack of energy. So it is only natural that thoughts of mortality flash through our minds during treatment and beyond.

These thoughts occur randomly and, of course, are not planned sessions to ponder death. Something as simple as a television program, movie, song on the radio, or innocent comment from a friend may trigger these reflections on death. It comes across your mind on a regular basis, perhaps monthly, perhaps weekly. This is a naturally occurring part of living with this disease. It is human nature to reflect on who we are, where are we going, what we are trying to accomplish on Earth, how will we die, and, most importantly, when will we die. This is not something that just happens to cancer patients but to all of us. The difference, obviously, is that cancer certainly makes the focus and the intensity sharper and, not to mention, the frequency much more often!

It is therefore necessary to acknowledge whatever statistics there are for your given cancer, but do not let it monopolize all your waking thoughts. Take this situation and make it a source of opportunities! Cancer is not the end of life, but the beginning of a new life. Certainly this disease focuses on death and mortality, but the last time I checked, we all have been told we would die some day anyway! Life is not forever. What seems to be the most important thing is how we live our life, no matter how long or how short.

The very challenge of cancer, in my humble opinion, is to allow the focus that diagnosis quickly brings to life to be a wake-up call to live the rest of your life to the fullest, whether it be six weeks or sixty years. Do what you want and like to do. Notice the small things around you, like the birds outside your window, the butterfly flitting in the flowerbed, the happy, blue sky, or even the deep, gray sky of a threatening storm. Smell the roses. You may have cancer, but no one can take away your joy of life! Make sure you have fun in your daily living. Look for humor in every day; it is just everywhere, if you look! Make someone smile. Do something nice for someone, or maybe just be nice for a change! Make your life a commitment to help make the world a better place in whatever way you can.

This might mean looking at things differently in your own little neighborhood or taking up the call on a much larger scale. It doesn't matter how big or small; just do what you can with whatever energy you have. If you *want* to do this, and if you have a positive attitude, you can take mortality and put it in its place. Your life can go on, even during treatment, and like the old Frank Sinatra song, you will be able to say, "I did it my way!" Make it the positive-attitude path.

One can actually become more energized with the right attitude! If we languish in the negativity of dwelling on our mortality, we will only start to feel sorry for ourselves and undoubtedly become depressed. What is key is taking the view that cancer is a challenge to us to make the most out of our lives. It is not so important how *long* we live but *how* we live!

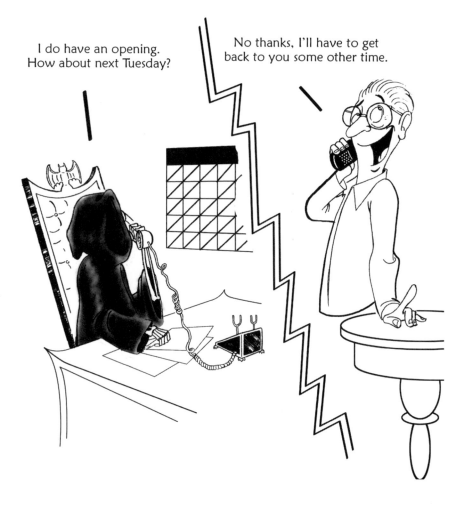

While coming to grips with mortality is part of the cancer scene, you must not allow those thoughts to overshadow daily life. You have to put it in perspective and focus on developing the attitude that there is so much to life. Make goals of the things you want to do and the places you want to go. What you want may be very elaborate or the simplest thing. After all, cancer tends to bring into the limelight the simplest things around us. Enjoy these things more than ever. The most important thing to accomplish is to make the most of every day to the greatest extent you can physically handle. This is the time to pack as much into your day as your body allows—*carpe diem* (seize the day)!

Courage

Dealing with mortality brings up the idea of courage. Whenever our mortality is brought into focus, we instinctively want to survive, and there is a natural courage in all of us to carry on in this struggle. However, sometimes a challenge to life can be very direct, and our minds can overemphasize the prospect of death rather than the need for survival. That is why courage is important—it allows us to face challenges while maintaining a positive attitude. We need tools to battle cancer and build a positive outlook. When we have these tools in hand, we have a means to survive.

So in this regard, given the diagnosis of a life-threatening disease and the inevitable thoughts of mortality that follow, you must gather as much courage as possible. It is very challenging to deal with it all. First, you must deal with the shock of diagnosis and the denial phase and then, move immediately into treatment, which can be very physically and mentally draining. During all of this, you must, as soon as possible, get a handle on your emotional and psychological frame of mind. For even the strongest of us, this can be a fearsome task, which is why, as a cancer patient, you have to have a healthy dose of courage.

On some days, it takes courage even to talk about cancer. The best of us will have days where it is emotional to think about aspects of cancer and life. Thinking about dying carries with it large amounts of feelings. To be able to talk about your cancer requires the courage to express your emotions and feelings to others. For most of us, the issues of major illness and death have not been particularly dwelled upon prior to cancer. To talk to others about it takes courage on a daily basis! There is often a great deal to overcome in discussing your emotions, but it is not impossible by any means. You have no choice but to bring out your feelings so that you can move on, and it takes a lot of courage to do this.

It is worth noting that talking about one's emotions and personal feelings is often much harder for men. It is largely a result of our society stereotyping males as "pillars of strength" who are not to show signs of weakness. Ironically enough, in situations like this, when discussing our emotions is important, men need extra strength and courage to overcome the very stereotype that expects it of them in the first place! It is much better for the patient, whether male or female, to get all of these feelings out, rather than keep them bottled up inside.

Courage is significant to a cancer patient; there is no denying it. Cancer forces us to tackle the tough issues and requires all our courage and strength. Overcoming these difficulties will boost your confidence and improve your attitude. Muster your courage, focus on your life ahead, and move forward!

> "The gem cannot be polished without friction,
> nor man perfected without trials."
> Chinese proverb

> "And in the end it's not the years in your life that count;
> it is the life in your years."
> Abraham Lincoln

CHAPTER 10
FEAR OF RECURRENCE

"The way I see it, if you want the rainbow, you gotta put up with the rain."
Dolly Parton, singer and actress

"We cannot direct the wind but we can adjust the sails."
Author unknown

For the majority of cancer patients, mortality is the main concern and remission the main goal. Even when remission is achieved, concern still lingers in the form of the possibility of recurrence. For most survivors, this concern is not all consuming, but it certainly remains in the back of our minds. Dealing with relapse in your primary cancer or even taking on a new cancer brings back all the anxieties that came with the original diagnosis. It is, in effect, reliving the ordeal all over again. So it is not unreasonable for cancer survivors—already very aware of and sensitive to changes in our bodies after having gone through the treatment process—to become very concerned at the slightest lump, faintest change in skin color, or most minute new ache or pain. And for those of us who monitor key numbers from blood tests, x-rays, and other pertinent markers, any change going the wrong direction will also spark concern. The fear of recurrence is a natural part of life as a cancer survivor, but you must learn to cope with it in ways that do not undermine but rather reinforce your positive attitude.

From a medical standpoint, there are several factors affecting the recurrence of cancer or the occurrence of a secondary cancer. For one, the type of cancer plays a big part. Some types of cancers are more prone to relapse, while others are not. Treatment for the primary cancer type and individual general health could also affect when or if a relapse will occur. Also, the stage of the first cancer will affect the possibility of a recurrence. The more advanced the cancer was the first time, the higher the probabilities of it coming back. The first step in a healthy defense against the fear of recurrence is to search out information specific to your situation and, with the help of your oncologist, to develop a routine that will put you in the best position to avoid recurrence.

A recent abstract from the Mayo Foundation for Medical Education and Research entitled "When Cancer Returns: How to Cope with Cancer Recurrence" talks about how recurrence can bring back many of the emotions you experienced in your first diagnosis. There is distress from "the shock of having the cancer come back after you assumed it was gone." Self-doubt may arise from questioning your judgment with previous treatment. The article states, "It is very common and reasonable to be angry that your cancer has returned. You might even be angry with your doctor for not stopping your cancer the first time." Finally, fatigue can arise from the stress of dealing with cancer again.

In coping with both the fear of recurrence and any actual recurrence, it is important to use the lessons learned from your first cancer experience. All the coping skills and support networks you used the first time should be brought to bear, and all the tools used to create and sustain a positive attitude should be employed. Positive attitude means that we have acknowledged our adversity and bad news and that we move on because we have so much to live for and accomplish. Whether it is the first cancer or the second (or even the hundredth for that matter!), the game plan is still the same: keep a positive attitude and go forward.

There are many advantages from the first go-around with cancer. Chances are that it would not be as difficult as the first time. You have been through the experience once, you already have established relationships with a medical team, you have adjusted your life to treatment before, and it is important to remember that you *did* get through it the first time. You may feel more control the second time. After all, you are

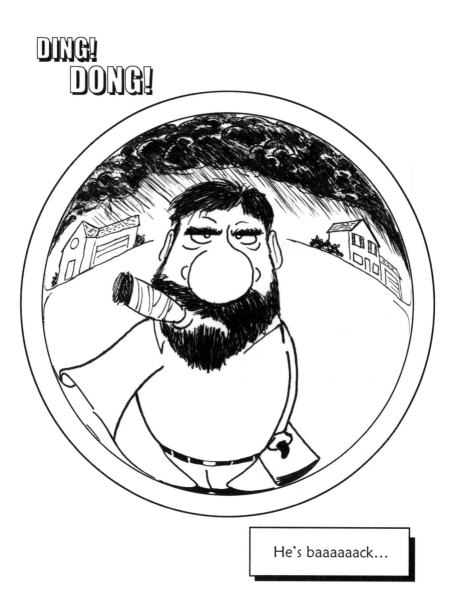

an experienced fighter! You have ready contacts, if you relapse, for a caregiver, support groups, and many other resources. Humor should always serve to ease recurrence. Certainly the power of your faith and religious beliefs will always carry you forward and, if anything, would be stronger than before.

Coping with recurrence is also much easier if you have developed some kind of exercise habits to keep your mind and body in reasonably good shape. This will continue to help through treatment if cancer does return. Along these lines, eating right always helps with your general health and your ability to handle treatment.

Preventive measures since your first cancer are in place. You probably are going to a doctor regularly for monitoring and follow-up care. Chances are that through regular office visits and ongoing treatment, any recurrence that may appear can be noted very early.

You must also remember that cancer research is improving, and advances are occurring every day. In fact, even the rate of progress in treating cancer is increasing each year. Since your first cancer, more options are available, and much has been done with new therapies to increase effectiveness and reduce side effects. As a result, survival rates are improving.

The road of life is full of bumps and hills. The fear of recurrence is just another bump, and actual recurrence, if it ever comes, would just be another hill to climb. All our positive attitude skills will serve us as we ride on in this new challenge in our path. The most important thing is that we live our life to the fullest and not let the possibility of recurrence consume our energies.

> "A bend in the road is not the end of the road . . .
> unless you fail to make the turn."
> Author unknown

> "To fear is one thing. To let fear grab you by
> the tail and swing you around is another."
> Katherine Paterson, author

CHAPTER 11
EXERCISE FOR MIND AND BODY

"Physical fitness is not only one of the most important keys to a healthy
body, it is the basis of dynamic and creative intellectual activity."
John F. Kennedy

P hysical exercise of any kind, aside from strengthening your body,
will also help your mind and improve your outlook during cancer.
For that matter, exercise is good regardless of who you are. There
are many articles and books everywhere about the benefits of exercising;
just ask your doctor! For patients dealing with cancer, it is more important than ever to try to move around and keep fit as best as possible.
The stress of dealing with doctor appointments, testing, chemotherapy,
biopsies, waiting for lab results, fatigue, physical pain, IVs, blood tests,
and radiation—these all take their toll. Exercise will clear the mind and
greatly help to give you a fresh attitude. If you have ever done any exercise—even something as simple as taking a walk outside—you know
how the fresh air and activity clear your mind. Better yet, many types of
exercise, such as walking, canoeing, and biking, also provide the needed
time to talk to a caregiver, spouse, or friend. In general, exercise, of any
type or at any level, will energize you to think better and feel better about
yourself and your day. You don't have to be a cancer survivor to benefit
from exercise!

There are numerous studies expounding the benefits of exercise
for cancer patients. For example, in the May 1, 1997 issue of *Cancer*,
the American Cancer Society reported a study in which one group of

cancer patients was given a supervised aerobic exercise program, while the other group had no particular program. Those cancer patients in the exercise group "experienced better physical performance, increased hemoglobin levels, and less fatigue than patients who did not exercise." A second study reported by the American Cancer Society showed that patients participating in two ten-week sessions of a wellness program that included aerobic exercise, strength training, flexibility, and relaxation, exhibited "a 43 percent increase in strength and a 50 percent increase in endurance." An even more recent study by the Dana-Farber Cancer Institute concluded that "colon cancer patients engaging in moderate levels of exercise six to twelve months after completing therapy had an approximately 50 percent higher survival rate than those who did not exercise." I could go on listing more and more studies, but the point is simple: exercise—even a little bit of it—has a considerable positive effect on cancer patients (and everybody else!).

Exercise relieves the stress in your body and provides a positive boost to your mind. You will feel better about yourself and everything around you. It will put an upbeat spin on your mind-set and spur you on with renewed energy to do other things. Your mind will be freer. You can set little goals with exercise and, over time, will find achievement in the ability to do better at your exercise. For example, you might not be able to run a marathon (few of us can!), and depending on your treatment and health, you may even have difficulty walking around the block. Do not let that dissuade you—walk only as far as you can, and then set a goal of going just a few feet farther the next day. Eventually, you will be able to do longer walks, go on longer bike rides, kick up the level adjustment on a fitness machine, or do more laps in the pool. Whatever it is, you will have a sense of accomplishment that comes with making your body do something it hasn't done before.

No matter what exercise you come up with, make sure you do what you like to do, and, if you are daring, try some new things. There are so many things to do; just pick the ones you like. There is walking, hiking, running, biking, aerobics classes, skiing, swimming, gardening, tennis, kayaking, cross country skiing, and more and more and more! On a tamer level, consider yoga, tai chi, or pilates as alternatives. If you are more of an indoor type, try the local YMCA or a commercial fitness center. Check out your local community center to see what classes they offer. I had always wanted to take a yoga class for the stretching and flexibility aspects, so I took a beginning class in yoga, which turned out to be really good for me. The best part of nearly every exercise class is that you can do them at your own pace and ability, and the movements can be modified to fit your energy, strength, and conditioning level. Some people can do more, and others can tone down their exertion or stretching according to how their body responds.

Of course, it is important to monitor yourself so that you do not overdo it. Exercise must be done within what your doctor and your body allow, but generally that can be a pretty wide array of choices. Do what you feel you can do, and just as importantly, do what you like to do. About once per week, I get in the pool at the YMCA and do some swimming, which is a great all-around exercise. I enjoy biking so I also go to the YMCA, especially in colder months, to ride the newer stationary bikes that allow you to check your heart rate, as well as set your level and length of workout. These types of machines allow you to monitor your workout as you advance. I also do some light weightlifting at the various stations that work other muscle groups besides the legs. I enjoy this exercise regimen because it is a nice combination of muscle toning and cardiovascular work (and aside from that, it's a lot of fun!).

In warmer weather, I am out on bike rides occasionally with two or three friends who also enjoy biking. These rides are done at a pace that fits the entire group. In pre-cancer years, they were longer and were used as training rides for the MS150 Bike Tour that I mentioned earlier in the book. For years, I participated in the MS150 Bike Tour in my home state of Michigan. This is an event sponsored in many states to raise money for the National Multiple Sclerosis organization. You basically pedal seventy-five miles on a Saturday and do the return seventy-five miles on Sunday. It is a great event: good exercise, a great cause, friendly people, and very well organized. I am very proud to say that through my participation I have raised more than twenty thousand dollars over the years!

Speaking of which, fundraisers for charities are wonderful sources of exercise. There are quite a few of these events, which typically are walks, runs, or rides. There are many different ones sponsored by all sorts of organizations with worthy causes. Keep your eyes open, and you will see flyers at malls, local stores, libraries, sporting stores, etc. These events are especially enjoyable and worthwhile because they combine three essential elements of building a positive attitude—exercise, volunteerism, and social interaction. I strongly recommend that you seek out these excellent opportunities. They give you a chance to help others, meet new people, and all the while, you exercise!

In addition to physical exercise, find areas where your mind can be

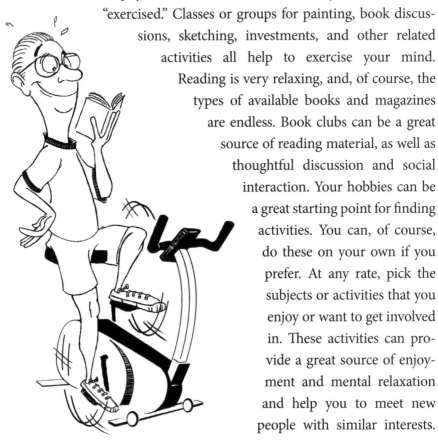

"exercised." Classes or groups for painting, book discussions, sketching, investments, and other related activities all help to exercise your mind. Reading is very relaxing, and, of course, the types of available books and magazines are endless. Book clubs can be a great source of reading material, as well as thoughtful discussion and social interaction. Your hobbies can be a great starting point for finding activities. You can, of course, do these on your own if you prefer. At any rate, pick the subjects or activities that you enjoy or want to get involved in. These activities can provide a great source of enjoyment and mental relaxation and help you to meet new people with similar interests.

These types of classes and special interest groups have many benefits: they increase your knowledge and skills, build your confidence, inspire you, and most importantly, restore a sense of achievement in your life.

I have also found that writing is a very good healing and relaxation technique. The best way to do this is to keep a journal. Whenever you feel the need during the week, open your journal and write whatever flows that day. The topics may be random, but that's okay. Your mind just needs to get out on paper your feelings, thoughts, and ideas. In effect, journaling is another way to get things off your mind and feed a positive attitude. There is relief to your mind through writing. You might even consider joining a writing or journaling class in your community or through a support group such as Gilda's Club or a cancer center.

It is great to get exercise, but it is even more helpful to do your exercise, both physical and mental, with someone who has the same interests. Your spouse or a friend can accompany you, and the exercise is much more enjoyable. You have someone to talk to, and, more importantly, you can motivate each other to be diligent about regular workouts. When someone is in your driveway waiting for you to go to the gym, it is hard to say you are not going to exercise! Find an exercise buddy!

The main point is to get out and do as much as you can. For some people, going to the mailbox is a major accomplishment, and still for others, it is running a marathon. What is challenging for us depends on our situation. It is important to monitor yourself so that you do not overdo it. Treat yourself carefully; you are or have been going through a demanding treatment regimen. Your body will tell you if it is being pressed too hard. Listen to your body, and enjoy the workout! Choose activities that you enjoy and find interesting. You will meet some interesting people, and I guarantee you will feel much better, both mentally and physically. Exercising provides healing for your body and mind and the whole you. You will feel better about yourself, and you will definitely have a more positive attitude.

"Lack of activity destroys the good condition of every human being, while movement and methodical physical exercise save it and preserve it."
Plato, philosopher

"Too many people confine their exercise to jumping to conclusions, running up bills, stretching the truth, bending over backward, lying down on the job, sidestepping responsibility, and pushing their luck."
Author unknown

CHAPTER 12
THE PATH TO A GOOD ATTITUDE: HUMOR

"A keen sense of humor helps us to overlook the unbecoming,
understand the unconventional, tolerate the unpleasant, overcome the
unexpected, and outlast the unbearable."
Billy Graham, evangelist

By far one of the most important factors for getting through cancer (and a lot of other things) is a good sense of humor. Though dealing with a life-threatening disease would not initially provoke one to laugh, it will greatly help to heal your mind along the way. Humor is a tension reliever. It takes the edge off an otherwise serious situation. A sense of wit is good for the mind and soul. There is so much seriousness about this disease that humor can cut through the tension and relax a patient greatly.

Here is an illuminating statement from the American Cancer Society's humor therapy materials: "Although available scientific evidence does not support claims that laughter can cure cancer or any other disease, it can reduce stress and enhance a person's quality of life. Humor has physical effects because it

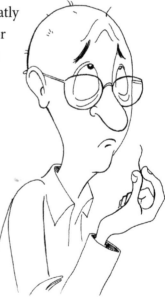

When cancer gets frustrating, you can't even pull your hair out!

can stimulate the circulatory system, immune system, and other systems in the body." In fact, the above statement really isn't necessary to make my point—the fact that the American Cancer Society even has something called "humor therapy" should tell you all that you need to know!

An article in the January 20, 2005 *Journal of Clinical Oncology* titled "Humor and Oncology" states that humor is "acknowledged to be a mature defense mechanism." It goes on to discuss how humor can help with the doctor-patient relationship by "setting the tone for a more relaxed atmosphere" and adds that "humor has an important role in establishing these relationships by breaking the ice, reducing the fear of the unfamiliar, and encouraging a sense of trust." A second report, conducted at Texas A & M University, found that humor is "a legitimate strategy for relieving stress and maintaining a general sense of well-being while increasing a person's hope." Again, I could go on naming studies, but it should suffice to say that, medically speaking, humor and laughter are good for you.

When patients have a sense of humor and can sometimes laugh at themselves, they will have a very positive affect also on their family, friends, and everyone else around them. If you can appreciate humor, others will certainly enjoy the humor with you, and it will cut through the tension, especially at the hardest times. This is particularly noticeable when you first talk to someone after they just found out about your diagnosis. If you display a sense of lightness, at least on some issues, they are much more relaxed and comfortable approaching you, knowing that you have not let death and darkness prevail over all your thoughts. You have effectively said, "I know I have cancer and all the complications that come with it, but I also know it will not stop me, and I will proceed on my life's path in spite of it!"

If you will indulge me, I would like to tell a personal story about my journey with cancer. I was just a few days out from diagnosis and was home with my newly inserted Groshong catheter. This, as many of you might know, is a small tube that is surgically inserted into your upper chest/clavicle area. It is inserted into the main artery going into the heart, and the other end comes out of your chest and hangs down about three or four inches. To keep it sterile, saran wrap–like patches are used that seal the catheter to your chest.

Well, I took my first shower after the surgery, and unluckily enough, there was a small gap on the top of the patch, which allowed water to seep in. This, of course, was obvious after the shower, as I now had water sloshing about inside my sterile patch! Great, I thought, another unforeseen challenge in my cancer journey. After deliberating for several minutes about how to solve this problem, my brilliant plan was to lean over the bathroom sink and simply allow the water to flow out. Great idea, but it didn't work; as hard as I tried, I could not lean over the sink far enough to let it drain out.

At that point, my wife, Jan, came into the room. Naturally, she was a little perplexed as to why her husband was bent double over the bathroom sink with a plastic pouch of water stuck to his chest. After I explained the predicament, she laughed and commiserated with me. Then she had her own great idea.

Jan told me to lie face up on the edge of the bed. Then she had me inch my way off the bed until my head and chest were hanging over the edge. Unfortunately, the pouch still wasn't draining, so I had to slide farther and farther off the bed. Finally, hanging so far off the bed that my wife had to hold my legs to keep me from crashing to the floor, bracing myself with my hands in a rather poor imitation of a headstand, I felt the water begin to drain. Sure, some of it might have drained up my nose, and sure, Jan said that my face turned bright red from all the blood rushing to it, but by golly, we were able to solve the problem!

I was sure that I did not remember reading about anything like this in the literature from my doctor, so I told him the story at my next appointment. I lamented to him that, despite all our modern technology, there wasn't an easier way to solve this problem. He laughed at my story (probably thinking, "Wait until I tell my buddies this one!") and said, "Of course there is an easier way." He then explained—very simply, I might add—how you can cover the patch with a Ziploc bag during showers. Even easier, he said, is to have a few extra patches available at home! As you might imagine, we all had a pretty good chuckle about it. It would have been easy for us to get embarrassed or bent out of shape about things like that, but we were able to keep our sense of humor throughout the cancer trip, and it has made a big difference.

In fact, pretty much everyone I told the story to laughed about it. It was one of those very practical, everyday problems that can come up with patients, but Jan and I somehow found a ridiculous approach to dealing with it. I can only imagine some of the stories that doctors and nurses hear from patients as they go through their week!

I, like most cancer patients, lost all my hair after chemotherapy and radiation. Even though it is stylish today for some men to have a shaved head, I found that "bald is beautiful" was not for me. At three months post-chemo, my hair was about one-eighth of an inch long, and I felt encouraged that I would have hair again. At this time, my youngest daughter was dating a boy who wore his hair all spiked with gel, as was common then. On one of his visits to the house, I told him that I would like to know the brand of gel he was using so that I could use it too. At first, he was a bit confused since there was nothing to gel on my head! But when he finally realized that I was joking, he thought it was hilarious.

Humor not only helps us as cancer survivors but also makes others around us feel better. I think we all have experienced the contagious effect of laughing. Once someone starts telling jokes or using humor in conversation, others usually jump in, and the enjoyment gets even better. It seems that humor rubs off, and, more importantly, people really prefer a light conversation and are easily attracted to humor. Everyone enjoys a good joke!

A great example of cancer patients keeping a sense of humor about themselves is "chemo-brain." Cancer patients often experience some memory loss during treatment, and we refer to this condition as chemo-brain. Apparently, there is some scientific and medical basis for this, as it is believed that we really do lose brain cells and some cognitive ability due to chemotherapy treatment. At support groups and in conversations with other survivors, we sometimes joke about how nice it is to be able to blame chemotherapy for short-term memory lapses whenever you want and get away with it! So the next time you cannot remember something or it slipped your mind, just take the "get out of jail free" card and declare that you have chemo-brain—just promise not to tell anyone our secret!

Laughter is good for the soul. There is no denying the healing quality of humor in our lives. I am sure we all have experienced how much we feel better and how our outlook improves after enjoying a good laugh. Not only should you enjoy good jokes, but you must also seek out humor

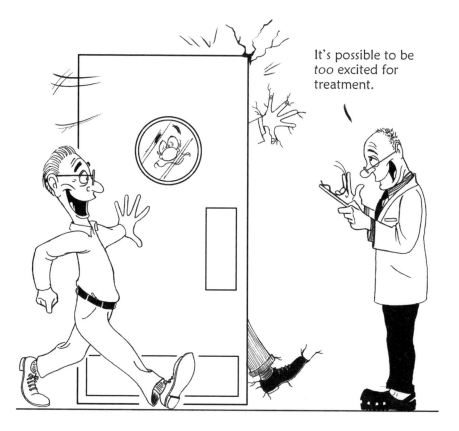

It's possible to be *too* excited for treatment.

wherever you can. Find a good sitcom on television, rent a funny movie (my all-time favorite is *Airplane!*), or try going to a comedy club. Don't forget to find humor in your daily life. It is there, just look for it!

Life should be fun! Take time to keep a light side to everyday living. Humor is one of the cancer survivor's greatest resources for a positive attitude. I guarantee you that there will be situations of your own that will undoubtedly be funny. Humor relieves the tension, makes things more bearable, and is enjoyed by most everyone. It will promote a positive attitude and will feed upon itself. Many times, a positive attitude will allow you simply to laugh at something rather than be so serious or tense about it. So lighten up and feel more relaxed—life is too short to have things so somber. Seek out humor and laugh often!

"Optimism and humor are the grease and glue of life.
Without both, we would never have survived our captivity."
Philip Butler, Vietnam prisoner of war

CHAPTER 13
THE BIGGER PICTURE:
VIEW OF THE WORLD

"Become a possibilitarian. No matter how dark things seem to be
or actually are, raise your sights and see the possibilities—
always see them, for they're always there."
Norman Vincent Peale, clergyman, author

Your view of the world around you is extremely critical to your attitude. In fact, perception is really just another measure of your attitude. When we talk about how we view things, we are talking about our day-to-day, hour-to-hour perspective. We are talking about the type of "eyeglasses" you use to look at your surroundings, and on a bigger scale, what you see for your role and future in life.

When a cancer patient gets up in the morning, what are the first thoughts about the day? Are they ones of disinterest, boredom, lack of enthusiasm, or depression? Or does the patient wake up full of energy to get started on the many activities planned for the day? The first feelings and thoughts about the day are the best indicators of a person's attitude. When your mind is clear as you open your eyes, what is the first thought that comes into your head? That is the defining moment that indicates where your attitude is positioned! Certainly we cannot be one-hundred-percent positive every single day upon waking. We all have days, no matter who we are, when we just aren't feeling good. Cancer patients may have days where they wake up with extra pain or discomfort due to treatments or just due to side effects of their disease. The ability to be chipper and ready to go is much more of a challenge on those days!

The more important issue is *what are you going to do with the day?* Are you going to feel sorry for yourself and dwell on all your aches and pains? Do you feel life is unfair and you have been cheated out of something? In other words, are you letting all the negatives overwhelm your life? Once again, is the glass half full or half empty?

You must realize that you have the power to change how you look at things on a daily basis. It is *your own choice* how you go forward; you make the decision for yourself. So are you approaching the day believing you will make the most of it, even though you might not be at your peak physically? Do you believe that there are so many things that you need to accomplish or places to go that you need to get up and get things done? Do you believe that life is too important to waste time and dwell on doom and gloom?

Which of the above scenarios describes your early morning thought waves? Even given that we all have "off days," what do you feel toward life on a regular basis? Are you often feeling down and short changed, or are you full of life and wanting to grab as much as you can every day? This is the fundamental issue at hand. What kind of view do you have through your set of "eyeglasses"?

If you suspect that you might be one of those who view the world as a half-empty glass, you need to turn your mind around. Reality is what you make it! Take that half-full glass and fill it the rest of the way. Live every day to the fullest of your abilities!

On weaker days, it takes a conscious effort, and therefore it must be our goal to feel good about ourselves. We must believe we have many things to contribute and accomplish in our lives. We have family and friends with whom we can do many things yet in our lives. And on a much bigger scale, the world is in need of many things to make it a better place.

There are many examples around us of people with cancer who proved that we are much more capable than we realize. These cancer survivors show us that all things are possible and that cancer does not limit who we are or what we are capable of achieving.

Lance Armstrong was given low odds for survival when he was diagnosed with cancer in his early twenties. After substantial treatment, he was healed and continued on from where he left off with his world-class cycling efforts. The rest is history as they say: he went on to win a record number of Tour de France races. What an outstanding example of determination, focus, and attitude for cancer survivors!

Barbara Hillary, an eight-year lung cancer survivor, is another wonderful example for us. Barbara skied to the North Pole. That in itself is a great accomplishment, but even more impressive is that she accomplished this feat at the age of 75. Furthermore, she had never skied in her life before deciding to tackle the North Pole. Barbara has an unstoppable attitude and always views the world as full of opportunities. In addition to her North Pole adventure, Barbara has also tried such adventures as dog sledding and polar bear photography.

While both the Lance Armstrong and Barbara Hillary stories are extreme examples of success of determination and attitude in the face of cancer, they both exemplify the idea of a very positive view of the world. We all may not be able to match these feats as cancer survivors, but the point is to take on the world to whatever level you can. Do not let cancer stop you from accomplishing as much as your mind and body can accept. Look around you in your world, and you will see many examples of people who, in spite of cancer, do great things in their lives.

The target for all of us should be to take the "flip side" view of the world. Whenever we find ourselves not being positive, we need to flip how we look at events, others, and our actions in order to create a more constructive direction. In other words, if we focused too much on the negative or downside in the past, we now need to think about how something positive can come from a turn of events. Life will be filled with both bad and good news. We must take bad news for what it is and keep on going at life with all the gusto we can muster. Look for ways to find the upside in all the events affecting your daily life, and remember the popular advice, "Life is not a bed of roses."

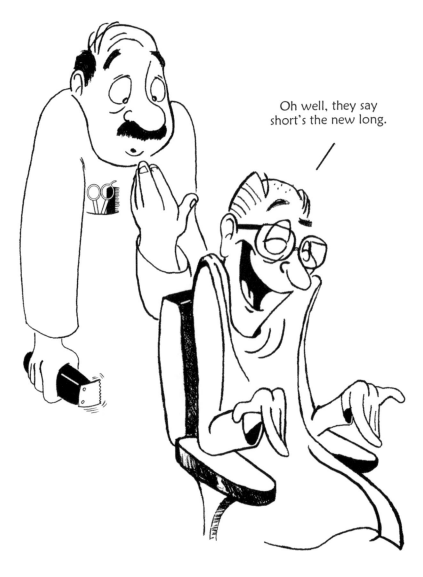

It takes time, focus, and practice to instill in your mind this ability to look for positive aspects in what appears to be bad news. The first step is to identify what, on initial perspective, looks like bad news. For example, say a support group meeting date comes up, and you really do not feel like you want to go out and talk about this disease. At this point, you must recognize that you are focusing on the negative aspect of the situation. Next, you must try to find the "flip side." Say to yourself, I know I will be better off going to the meeting and just checking out what others have to say. Consider the possibility that you will learn something of interest to your situation. Undoubtedly, what happens is that you will find more than you thought you would, end up talking more about your situation than you thought you wanted to, and will probably meet some new and interesting patients. All of these people are trying to deal with cancer. You will find ways that help you deal with it too!

I would be lying if I told you that it will be easy to live with cancer, but recognize it for what it is. We have to work through therapy and protocol and focus on recovery so we can accomplish the many things we want to do. As we go through it all, we must make the best of the rest of our lives, for however long we are destined to be here. The world awaits our contribution! Enjoy the time you have.

If you work at it every day, you will see what can be accomplished by changing your outlook and seeking the positive in each situation. Your positive attitude will permeate your life, thoughts, and actions. It will feed on itself and become contagious to others around you. Your positive attitude will buoy everyone's spirits. You will become an inspiration to others!

"I take nothing for granted. I now have only good days or great days."
Lance Armstrong, seven-time Tour de France winner

"They can conquer who believe they can."
Virgil, Roman poet

CHAPTER 14
THE PATH TO A GOOD ATTITUDE: HOPE

"There is no medicine like hope, no incentive so great, and no tonic so powerful as expectation of something tomorrow."
O.S. Marden

In the final analysis, the biggest end result of a positive attitude is that we have hope. We should be filled and overflowing with hope! But what is hope? Hope is the belief in a positive future. It is the belief that good things will happen to us in the future. It is a statement that great things are ahead for us. Hope is a conviction that our lives, however long, will have served a purpose and impacted others around us. Because we have hope and a positive attitude, we are mentally prepared to handle adversity, we feel we can still contribute, and we are optimistic. We believe things happen in our lives for a reason. We see our contribution to the world around us as a higher goal. We do all we can to make our world a better place. It may be as simple as our immediate world of family and friends. It could also go even larger to our community and beyond. Our impact and reach with our attitude will go as far as we individuals want it to be. It is only limited by physical strength and our desire.

We all need hope, with or without cancer. It is important to all of life, but even more so in times of adversity. Hope brings out the best in all of us. The hope that we display inspires those we come into contact with on a daily basis. When we have a good attitude, hope is fueled. We are motivated to try harder and to do more in life.

Promote hope all around you. Start with little things and build from there. For example, make a phone call to a friend or check in on a cancer survivor. You can move on from there, by going to the store for someone who cannot get out. Doing things for others will provide hope for you and the friend. Also, there are things for your own well-being which you can do, such as sit in a garden and watch the birds. Absorb the beauty of a flower blooming. Feed your hobbies and interests. All these types of things provide hope and inspiration to your life and the lives of others.

We will have bumps in the road, and we may even fall off our bike along the way. That's life, but the most important thing is to *get back on the bike*. We need to continue the ride and be determined, because there is so much for us to see, to do, and to contribute, that we must squeeze as much as possible into our daily lives. We must live everyday to the max!

Hope is nourished by faith and religion. Indeed, our religious beliefs can create and reinforce hope within us. Those who have a belief in a higher being or a higher purpose will always have hope if they keep the faith. In fact, the whole premise of Christian life is that Christ has already given us an example of hope despite adversity by his dying on the cross and providing eternal life.

Throughout our journey, we must step back and count our blessings. We are more fortunate than maybe we realize! Over time we may have taken things for granted. We have so much to be thankful for: our families, our friends, our gardens, sunny days, home, a great country to live in, and the list goes on. Really think about your surroundings, and you will be amazed at how much you have. We probably didn't notice some of these blessings before cancer came, but they really are all around us.

Appreciating what I have was one of the biggest positives that came out of my cancer. My diagnosis provided the opportunity to really view differently what is important to me. As a result of the whole cancer experience, my focus has changed. What is important now tends to be more personal things, such as family. The focus has shifted away from career and work. Small things are much more appreciated. Simple things, such as gardening, provide an opportunity for me to appreciate nature.

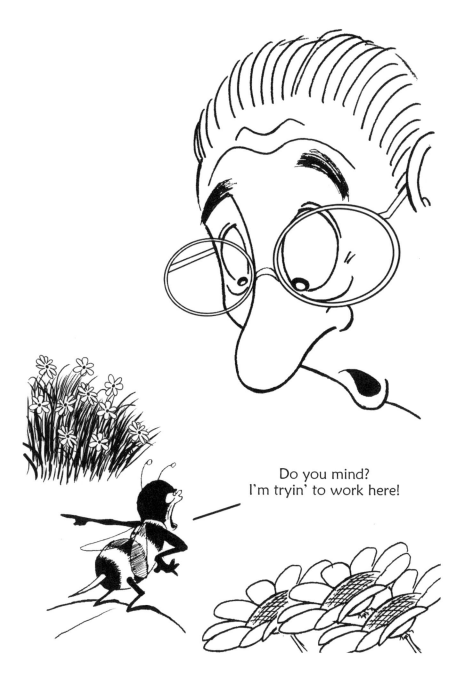

The plants, birds, butterflies, and insects that visit the garden provide an immense amount of gratitude for life's simple joys. For example, it amazes me when I truly take the time in the summer to watch the bees as they do their pollen collection. (Try, it and you'll see why we say "busy as a bee!") Yes, I actually watch them closely doing their jobs! Nature teaches us so much about living and how miraculous all God's creatures are. It may sound minute, but for me this is a main focus at this stage in life.

When we have appreciation for everything—from the simple fact that we are alive to all the little things in our lives—we build our hope beyond our immediate cancer concern. In fact, if we step back we should realize that adversity, even cancer, is a gift. It teaches us to be better human beings. We appreciate everything we have, starting with the opportunity to open our eyes each day. Cancer refocuses our attention to what is important. Hope provides an opportunity to travel a whole new road in life after hitting a bump of challenging times.

Life takes on new meaning from the hope that is out there. Hope is a powerful driver on a trip through adversity.

"Although the world is full of suffering, it is full also of the overcoming of it."
Helen Keller, author

CHAPTER 15
CONCLUSION:
REWARDS OF A POSITIVE ATTITUDE

"Enjoy the little things, for one day you may look back and realize they
were the big things."
Robert Brault, writer

I have attempted throughout the course of this book to show the way
toward a positive attitude. Cancer isn't easy. It has a dramatic impact
on us physically, mentally, and emotionally. Striving for as much of a
positive attitude as possible when coping with a life-threatening disease
is critical to making the most of the situation. Positive attitude works.

I have laid out in this book the many components that help build a
positive attitude, make your trip with cancer easier, and offer the potential for a deeper and stronger understanding of your life. We must be
the determined fighter and persevere in this struggle. A strong support system, including a caregiver, is essential. Gather information and
knowledge on your disease and treatment and talk about it with others.
The knowledge gained will greatly minimize the fear of the unknown. A
strong religious conviction and faith will give you strength throughout
the cancer journey and for your entire life going forward. Courage to
face all the challenges in life, including mortality and cancer recurrence, is essential to coping with adversity. Along the way, help yourself,
mentally and physically, by doing whatever level and form of exercise
works for you. It is important to use humor often, and it will help ease
the heaviness and make the trip fun! View the world and your life on

a bigger scale, and think about what you can contribute. Always have hope—believe that your life will be fuller with a positive attitude, and your life will have more meaning than ever.

Like cancer itself, there are no magical cures or easy solutions for most of this. However, it behooves all cancer survivors to make the most of what they have. It is the essence of life that we, as individuals, do all we can with our lives. Make the world a better place for having been here. The magnitude of our contribution may be limited to one or two people, or it may take on a global impact, or anything in between. The most important aspect is that every day we are living our lives to the utmost. One of my very favorite statements is what the U.S. Army used for its recruiting campaign a few years ago. It was simply, "Be all that you can be!" There is no other expression that defines our daily challenge as humans. It takes on a special need for those of us dealing with cancer. We must strive for the maximum on a daily basis, in our work, play, relationships, and betterment of the world. If we individually believe in being the best at whatever we do, we will collectively make things so much better. Our attitudes will serve as the driving force behind all that we accomplish. Our relationships with each other will be dramatically impacted for the better.

In psychology courses, they talk about Abraham Maslow's concept of the hierarchy of needs, sometimes called the self-actualization theory. Self-actualization has always intrigued me, and the theory became even more focused as I went through the cancer journey. The hierarchy of needs describes the fundamental needs of every human being, with the highest one being the need to develop the full potentialities of oneself. What it means for each of us will vary depending on our potentialities. For some it is being a leader in the community; for others, it is being a top scientist; and for still others, it simply means living your life fully. At the point of self-actualization, you are at the highest level of achieving your life goals and maximizing your abilities. This concept is worth striving for in our lives. It provides a very high goal for us individually. It, along with our attitude, can be a target to constantly strive for as a more complete mind and body experience. It raises the bar, so to speak, and sets out before us an optimum lifetime experience. Working toward self-actualization makes us more complete. Using it as a goal forces us to strive to be the best we can be and therefore provides us with a higher level of living. Consider thinking of your own process toward self-actualization as part of your goal of a positive attitude.

We cannot be "pumped" and positive every single day. We will have days when our energy levels are not as strong as other days. Treatment and our body will tell us to ease up for the day. Even the healthy individuals around us have off days. Every day with cancer cannot be perfect; nevertheless, we must do the best we can. It is okay to have days when you are not as cheery as others. However, if your goal is to have hope and a positive attitude, you will continue to try to do your very best each day. Keep riding on to your overall goal of a positive attitude. Keep the long-term view that the days ahead will be even better. Strive for days where you can take on the world. Above all, never give up!

Perhaps there will be a cure for the various cancers someday, and that day may not be too many years off. In the meantime, it is necessary for those of us affected by it to make the most of our lives. Life always has its ups and downs and its good days and bad days. That much is out of our control. But we do have a choice in the matter—we can journey through life feeling down, without hope, and feeling cheated, or we can take life's challenges and find a way to turn them into positives. Attitude is a *choice*—we can control it. The power to pick the path we ride is within each of us. Why not take the high road? Take the path with a smoother ride and better view. Look at things differently, look at things with a positive attitude, and look at problems as opportunities. If we have the choice, then we might as well spend the rest of our lives doing what we like to do and living life the best we can. We must be determined and passionate about reaching our goals and enjoying life. We need to contribute the most we can to the world with whatever talents and abilities we have. What we do may be simple or it may be complex, but it should be done with a desire to do the best we can. You do not want to get to the end of your life and say that you did not try. That would be a waste of human talent and individual uniqueness. In fact, because of cancer, you have the opportunity to be even more inspired and even more determined to contribute as much as you can. Life really can be short, and we all have abilities and experiences to share and utilize for the betterment of the world.

On a daily basis, no matter how hard things get, count your blessings. No matter who you are, you have many, and they are there in front of you. Take the time to truly look around, and you will see them. Whether you may have a wonderful family, a beautiful smile, a good heart to help others, a deep sense of faith in God, or a blooming flower in the garden, these are all blessings. Or if you think about it, we are so fortunate to be living in one of the greatest countries in the world. Find your blessings, they are there, and enjoy them every day. We should be in awe of all there is around us. They do not have to be big items, but what is important is to recognize and appreciate them. Gratitude for everything takes on a more important role for the cancer survivor. Survivors should find it all the more reason to be grateful due to cancer.

View cancer as a gift. It is a chance to look closely at your life. It is a new beginning to do even better things with your life. Cancer is a positive—it is the opportunity to create a new phase of your life! It is an opening to reassess who you are and where you are going. It is that "golden opportunity" to improve your life for the better. People around us are so special. God has put all these beautiful creatures around us. Each is unique and dearer than ever. It can only be God above who could have come up with such an infinite variety of things for us to ponder. We are truly blessed to have this opportunity to have a life on earth!

We need to be steadfast, focused, and committed to the path of feeling good about ourselves. Our goal should be to put every action, every activity, and every thought on a positive note. Perfection is not necessary (or even possible), but we must maintain the belief that ongoing attention to a positive attitude will carry us through. It is the desire to do better and to make the most of what we do have that is the most critical aspect.

Lastly, deliberately think about your daily situations as they arise. Actually stop to consider them, and visualize that there can be a positive side to most everything. While we all will have our ups and downs as we go through life, we can still develop a positive view of the world. Think about events in a more favorable way, rather than dwelling on the negative. This can be challenging if you are not used to it. It takes practice, and the main point is to view the upside in things. It is much like getting a new pair of eyeglasses that allow for a much clearer view of the world around us. Despite adversity and hard times, all things can work out in the end.

Use your positive attitude in cancer to get what I call that spine-tingling feeling. What I am talking about is a feeling of utter joy. You may realize on some days that all is right with the world despite everything going on around you. You feel that you are doing what you need to be doing in your life. You feel you are making a contribution in some way toward a better world. With all of this in mind, you get this tingle up and down your spine that elicits a feeling of joy and excitement. It is the ultimate positive in your life. Keep a positive attitude as your goal, and you will get that same feeling. It is a confirmation that you are enjoying the ride of life.

I hope this book has helped you to develop a positive attitude. Maybe you picked up a tip, or maybe you learned many new things. Nurture your positive attitude. Work at it a little each day. The process is ongoing, but be determined to achieve the attitude that will carry you through this or any challenge. Have fun and enjoy life. Laugh often! Celebrate life no matter how much adversity comes your way. May God continue to bless you and guide you through your ride with cancer and all that comes after. And remember, this is the ride of your life!

"Whether you think you can or whether you think you can't, you are right."
Henry Ford

"Yesterday is gone. Tomorrow has not yet come.
We have only today. Let us begin."
Mother Theresa, religious leader

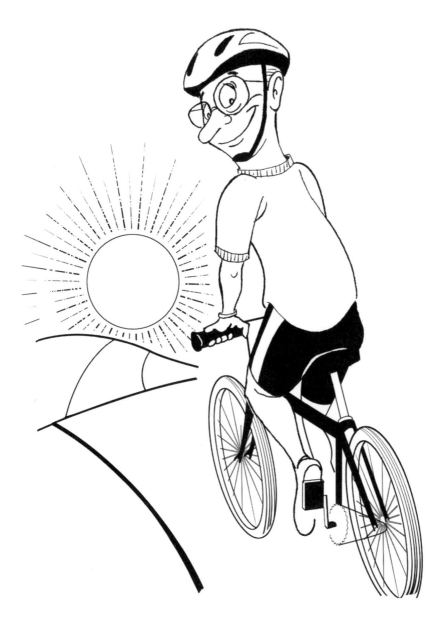

Acknowledgements

There are so many I'd like to thank who directly or indirectly helped make my dream of writing this book come true:

My wife, Jan, who more than tolerated the "time alone" sessions that I needed behind a closed door to allow me to write this book.

My three daughters, Christina, Carrie, and Cathy, and my son-in-law, Barron, who all gave encouragement along the way.

Jeff Covieo, whose wonderful illustrations brought my book to life.

A special thank you for those who were generous and courageous about sharing their adversity story for my Appendix III.

My publisher, Marian Nelson, and my editor, Ryan Schrauben, who worked with me to provide the publishing aspects of this book.

Father Brian Chabala, pastor of St. Fabian, who graciously took his time early on to read and critique the manuscript.

Dorothy Pitsch, an author of two books herself, who gave much encouragement for me to write, plus time explaining the publishing process.

And to those special people called cancer survivors, who I have met along the way in my cancer journey, thank you for helping me understand what it takes to be a survivor with a positive attitude.

APPENDIX 1
RESOURCES

ANEMIA:

**Aplastic Anemia & MDS
International Foundation, Inc.**
P.O. Box 310
Churchton, MD 20733
800-747-2820 or 410-867-0242
www.aamds.org
This organization is the oldest and largest patient advocate and support nonprofit for aplastic anemia, MDS, and other bone marrow diseases.

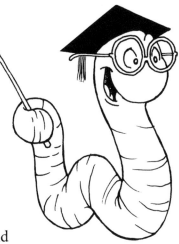

BLADDER CANCER:

Bladder Cancer Advocacy Network
888-901-BCAN (888-901-2226) or 301-215-9099
4813 St. Elmo Ave.
Bethesda, MD 20814
www.bcan.org
Strives to improve awareness and increase research for bladder cancer.

Bone Marrow/Stem Cell Transplant Information:

The Bone Marrow Foundation
337 East Eighty-Eighth St., Ste. 1B
New York, NY 10128
800-365-1336 or 212-838-3029
www.bonemarrow.org
This organization provides resources, information, programs, and services about bone marrow/stem cell transplantation.

Blood & Marrow Transplant Information Network (BMT Infonet)
2310 Skokie Valley Rd., Ste. 104
Highland Park, IL 60035
888-597-7674 or 847-433-3313
www.bmtinfonet.org
Publishes patient guides and a newsletter; links not only transplant patients with survivors, but all family members involved in the process as well; maintains a directory of transplant centers and helps with insurance problems.

National Bone Marrow Transplant Link (nbmtLINK)
20411 W. Twelve Mile Rd., Ste. 108
Southfield, MI 48076
800-546-5268 or 248-358-1886
www.nbmtlink.org
This organization has educational information, including booklets and a video, about bone marrow and stem cell transplants. Provides peer support to BMT patients and health professionals.

National Marrow Donor Program (NMDP)
3001 Broadway St. NE, Ste. 500
Minneapolis, MN 55413
800-MARROW-2 (800-627-7692)
Office of Patient Advocacy
888-999-6743
www.marrow.org

NMDP is funded by the federal government and keeps a registry of potential bone marrow donors, connecting patients, doctors, donors, and researchers to the resources they need to help more people live longer and healthier lives.

BRAIN TUMOR:

American Brain Tumor Association
2720 River Rd.
Des Plaines, IL 60018
800-886-2282 or 847-827-9910
www.abta.org
The ABTA provides information about brain tumors, new treatments, and help living with the diagnosis of a brain tumor.

Brain Tumor Society
124 Watertown St., Ste. 3H
Watertown, MA 02472
800-770-8287 or 617-924-9997
www.tbts.org
Provides free educational resources and individualized consultation for patients and families. The Brain Tumor Society sponsors educational symposia and conferences.

National Brain Tumor Foundation (NBTF)
22 Battery St., Ste. 612
San Francisco, CA 94111-5520
800-934-2873 or 415-834-9970
www.braintumor.org
NBTF provides information about coping with brain tumors. This organization also sponsors conferences, a medical advice nurse, and a newsletter. In addition, it raises funds for brain tumor research and provides caregivers with information and workshops.

BREAST CANCER:

breastcancer.org
7 E. Lancaster Avenue
Ardmore, PA 19003
www.breastcancer.org
Provides support with over two thousand pages of physician-reviewed breast cancer information on the internet, discussion boards, and a twenty-four-hour chat room.

National Alliance of Breast Cancer Organizations (NABCO)
9 E. Thirty-Seventh St., 10th Floor
New York, NY 10016
888-806-2226 or 212-889-0606
www.nabco.org
This organization maintains an online breast cancer resource list, which offers information for the patient regarding treatments, support, research, etc.

Sisters Network, Inc.
8787 Woodway Drive, Ste. 4206
Houston, TX 77063
866-781-1808 or 713-781-0255
www.sistersnetworkinc.org
Sisters Network focuses on increasing awareness of breast cancer in the African-American community, as well as providing individual and group support, education, advocacy, and research.

Susan G. Komen Breast Cancer Foundation
5005 LBJ Fwy., Ste. 250
Dallas, TX 75244
877-465-6636
www.komen.org
This is a tremendous source of breast cancer information and support. The Komen Breast Cancer Foundation is the sponsor of many fundraisers on a national basis and is dedicated to advancing research, treatment, and education for breast cancer. The foundation awards research grants annually.

Y-ME National Breast Cancer Organization, Inc.
212 W. Van Buren, Ste. 1000
Chicago, IL 60607
800-221-2141 or 312-986-8338
www.y-me.org
Y-ME provides information and support for breast cancer patients. They have a national 24/7 hotline and support group program. Services such as wigs and prostheses are provided for women with limited resources.

CANCER—GENERAL & SURVIVORSHIP:
(SEE ALSO MAGAZINE SECTION)

American Cancer Society (ACS)
1599 Clifton Rd. NE
Atlanta, GA 30329
800-227-2345 or 404-320-3333
www.cancer.org
The ACS provides a variety of research, printed information, and educational information for cancer patients and their families.

American Institute for Cancer Research (AICR)
1759 R St. NW
Washington, DC 20009
800-843-8114
www.aicr.org
AICR focuses on diet and nutrition as a way of preventing cancer.

Cancer Care, Inc.
275 Seventh Ave.
New York, NY 10001
800-813-4673 or 212-712-8400
www.cancercare.org
Cancer Care offers counseling, financial assistance, educational information, and practical help for cancer patients and their families, face to face, by telephone, and online.

Cancer Hope Network
Two North Rd., Ste. A
Chester, NJ 07930
877-HOPENET (877-467-3638) or 908-879-4039
www.cancerhopenetwork.org
This organization provides support by matching patients and their
families with volunteers who have faced cancer.

Cancer Research Institute
National Headquarters
One Exchange Plaza
55 Broadway, Ste. 1802
New York, NY 10006
800-99-CANCER (800-992-2623) or 212-688-7515
www.cancerresearch.org
The Cancer Research Institute focuses on research targeting
immunological methods for treating and preventing cancer.

Cancervive
6500 Wiltshire Blvd., Ste. 500
Los Angeles, CA 90048
310-203-9232
www.cancervive.org
Cancervive is dedicated to the challenge of life after cancer. This
nonprofit provides support, public education, and advocacy to
cancer survivors and their families.

Gilda's Club Worldwide
322 Eighth Ave., Ste. 1402
New York, NY 10001
888-445-3248
www.gildasclub.org
This very proactive organization was founded on behalf of Gilda
Radner. It is an international network where men, women, and
children with cancer and their families and friends join together
to build social and emotional support as a supplement to medical
care in a free, nonresidential, home-like setting. People with all

kinds and stages of cancer are welcome in thirty locations in the U.S. and Canada. Programs provided include, but are not limited to, networking groups, wellness groups, potlucks, lectures, various activities groups (art, yoga, color penciling, singing, etc.)—all with learning, sharing and fun in mind.

Lance Armstrong Foundation (LAF)
P.O. Box 161150
Austin, TX 78716
512-236-8820
www.livestrong.org
Helps people with cancer focus on living: unity is strength, knowledge is power, and attitude is everything. The LAF provides practical information and tools for cancer survivors and their families. It does this through advocacy, education, public health, and research efforts.

Medscape
www.medscape.com
This website provides regular email newsletters that cover a wide range of cancer topics including new drugs for cancer, new treatment protocols, clinical trials, and research findings on many types of cancers. The home site also has numerous topics and information on many general medical categories of interest.

National Cancer Institute (NCI)
6116 Executive Blvd.
Room 3036A
Bethesda, MD 20892
800-4-CANCER (800-422-6237)
www.cancer.gov
NCI provides a complete source for cancer patients for information on cancer, including disease descriptions, clinical studies, prevention, and links to cancer centers.

National Center for Complimentary and Alternative Medicine
9000 Rockville Pike
Bethesda, MD 20892
888-644-6266
www.nccam.nih.gov
The NCCAM provides the latest news, research, events, and
clinical trials involving complimentary medicine.

National Coalition for Cancer Survivorship
1010 Wayne Ave., Ste. 770
Silver Spring, MD 20910
877-NCCS-YES (877-622-7937) or 301-650-9127
www.canceradvocacy.org
NCCS offers support for cancer survivors and their families,
as well as information on cancer topics and a resource guide.
Additionally, the NCCS provides free CarePages.com for
individuals to set up their own private cancer website for
communication and support from others.

People Living With Cancer
888-651-3038 or 703-519-2927
www.plwc.org
This patient site provided by American Society of Clinical
Oncology contains guides for many types of cancer, as well as
guidance on coping, caregiving, and more.

CAREGIVERS:

Family Caregiver Alliance
180 Montgomery St., Ste. 1100
San Francisco, CA 94104
800-445-8106 or 415-434-3388
www.caregiver.org
This organization supports needs of families and friends who
provide long-term care at home.

National Family Caregivers Association
10400 Connecticut Ave., Ste. 500
Kensington, MD 20895
800-896-3650 or 301-942-6430
www.nfcacares.org
NFCA provides information, education, support, public awareness, and advocacy for caregivers.

Well Spouse Association
63 W. Main St., Ste. H
Freehold, NJ 07728
800-838-0879 or 732-577-8899
www.wellspouse.org
Provides support to wives, husbands, and partners of chronically ill and/or disabled persons.

CHILDREN:

Cancer Care for Kids
275 Seventh Ave., Floor 22
New York, NY 10001
800-813-HOPE (800-813-4673) or 212-712-8400
www.cancercareforkids.org
This organization offers online and telephone support groups, telephone education workshops, and online information.

Candlelighters Childhood Cancer Foundation
P.O. Box 498
Kensington, MD 20895
800-366-CCCF (800-366-2223) or 301-962-3520
www.candlelighters.org
This is a support organization for children with cancer and adult survivors. It provides information, support, and advocacy, and sponsors support groups, summer camps, and funding for those cancer patients in need.

Children's Brain Tumor Foundation (CBTF)
274 Madison Avenue, Ste. 1004
New York, NY 10016
866-228-4673
www.cbtf.org
Offers a free resource guide, *Parker's Brain Storm* (a book for children), the Parent-to-Parent Network, newsletter, annual teleconferences, and funds research.

The Children's Cancer Foundation, Inc.
1052 Flagtree Ln.
Baltimore, MD 21208
410-486-4744
www.childrenscancerfoundation.org
This foundation is committed to raising funds for many years for research and treatment of cancers affecting children.

Children's Cancer Research Fund (CCRF)
11633 San Vincente Blvd., Ste. 106
Los Angeles, CA 90049
310-207-5330
www.ccrf-kids.org
CCRF focuses on support for clinical research for children's cancers.

CureSearch National Childhood Cancer Foundation
4600 East West Hwy., Ste. 600
Bethesda, MD 20814
800-458-6223
www.CureSearch.org
CureSearch provides research data, information, and support to patients, survivors, family, and friends, based on a child's age, diagnosis, and treatment phase.

Kids Cancer Network
P.O. Box 4545
Santa Barbara, CA 93140
www.kidscancernetwork.org
The website contains a bimonthly "FUNLETTER" magazine resource center. A prayer network, a "your story" area, and Affection Connection certificates are available for medical caregivers.

Kids Konnected
27071 Cabot Rd., Ste. 102
Laguna Hills, CA 92653
800-582-5443 or 949-582-5443
www.kidskonnected.org
Kids Konnected provides friendship, education, summer camps, twenty-four-hour hotline, and support to kids who have a parent with cancer or have lost a parent to cancer.

The National Children's Cancer Society
One South Memorial Drive, Ste. 800
St. Louis, MO 63102
314-241-1600
www.children-cancer.org
This organization is focused on improving the quality of life for children with cancer by promoting children's health through financial and in-kind assistance, advocacy, support services, and education.

CLINICAL TRIALS:

CancerGuide
www.cancerguide.org
This website is maintained by a cancer survivor and features general cancer information in addition to information about participating in clinical trials.

CenterWatch
Twenty-Two Thomson Place, 47F1
Boston, MA 02210
617-856-5900
www.centerwatch.com
This company has an extensive list of approved clinical trials.

Coalition of National Cancer Cooperative Groups, Inc.
1818 Market St., Ste. 1100
Philadelphia, PA 19103
877-520-4457
www.cancertrialshelp.org
Research sponsored by the National Cancer Institute.

National Institutes of Health (NIH)
www.clinicaltrials.gov
This comprehensive website offers information on enrollment and
participation in clinical trials, as well as a searchable database of
current trials.

Oncolink
877-601-8601
www.oncolink.upenn.edu or www.emergingmed.com
This site contains extensive general cancer information and has
partnered the Abramson Cancer Center of the University of
Pennsylvania with EmergingMed.com to provide free matching
service for clinical trials.

PDQ Database
www.cancer.gov
This is the National Cancer Institute's database of clinical trials,
which can be sorted from 1,700 trials.

The Pharmaceutical Research and Manufacturers of America (PhRMA)
950 F Street, NW
Washington, DC 20004
202-835-3400
www.phrma.org
PhRMA represents the leading pharmaceutical and biotechnology companies in the U.S. The website provides information on new drugs being developed as well as a directory of prescription drugs and patient assistance programs.

The Association of Community Cancer Centers (ACCC)
11600 Nebel St., Ste. 201
Rockville, MD 20852
301-984-9496
www.accc-cancer.org
The Clinical Trials Resource Center offers access to the NCI PDQ database and an international database compiled by Thomson Center Watch, which provides information by state.

COLORECTAL CANCER:

C3: Colorectal Cancer Coalition:
1225 King St., 2nd Floor
Alexandria, VA 22314
703-548-1225
www.c-three.org
C3 promotes research to improve screening, diagnosis, and treatment of colorectal cancer.

Colon Cancer Alliance (CCA)
5411 N. University Dr., Ste. 202
Coral Springs, FL 33067
877-422-2030
www.ccalliance.org
The organization is comprised of colon and rectal cancer survivors

and their caregivers. Services provided include a buddy program, educational materials, clinical trial information, and news about colorectal cancer treatment and research.

Colorectal Cancer Network
P.O. Box 182
Kensington, MD 20895
301-879-1500
www.colorectal-cancer.net
This organization focuses on raising public awareness and finding information about colorectal cancers and also offers support services for colorectal patients.

ESOPHAGEAL CANCER:

Esophageal Cancer Awareness Association, Inc.
P.O. Box 25792
Tamara, FL 33320
www.ecaware.org
Provides support for esophageal cancer patients and caregivers.

FINANCIAL ASSISTANCE & FUNDRAISING:
(SEE ALSO PHARMACEUTICAL REIMBURSEMENT SECTION)

Children's Leukemia Foundation of Michigan
29777 Telegraph Rd., Ste. 1651
Southfield, MI 48034
800-825-2536 or 248-353-8222
www.leukemiamichigan.org
The Children's Leukemia Foundation provides information, financial assistance, and emotional support to families of adults and children affected by leukemia, lymphoma, and other blood disorders.

Chronic Disease Foundation
10880 Johm W. Elliot Dr., Ste. 400
Frisco, TX 75034
877-968-7233 or 972-712-0201
www.cdfund.org
The Chronic Disease Fund is a nonprofit organization with a focus on providing assistance to those under-insured patients who are diagnosed with chronic or life-altering diseases requiring use of expensive, specialty therapeutics.

Health Insurance Association of America
601 Pennsylvania Ave. NW
South Building, Ste. 500
Washington, D.C. 20004
202-778-3200
www.hiaa.org
This is an insurance-industry site that has links for consumers regarding finding insurance and types of policies.

National Transplant Assistance Fund
150 N. Radnor Chester Rd., Ste. F-120
Radnor, PA 19087
800-642-8399
www.transplantfund.org

NeedyMeds, Inc.
www.needymeds.com
The website provides a list of prescription assistance programs available from drug companies. Patients cannot apply directly to these programs. You need to have a doctor, nurse, or social worker contact NeedyMeds on your behalf.

Patient Access Network Foundation
P.O. Box 221858
Charlotte, NC 28222
866-316-PANF (866-316-7263)
www.patientaccessnetwork.org

The PANF is a charitable foundation dedicated to helping provide medication access to those with inadequate insurance.

Patient Advocate Coalition
www.patientadvocacy.net
This website provides links to cancer advocacy sites.

Patient Advocate Foundation (PAF)
700 Thimble Shoals Blvd., Ste. 200
Newport News, VA 23606
800-532-5274
www.patientadvocate.org
PAF provides education, legal counseling, and referrals to cancer patients and survivors on matters relating to health insurance, financial issues, job discrimination, and debt crisis.

HEAD AND NECK:

Support for People with Oral and Head and Neck Cancer, Inc. (SPOHNC);
P.O. Box 53
Locust Valley, NY 11560
800-377-0928
www.spohnc.org
Offers support and information addressing the emotional, psychological, and humanistic needs of oral, head, and neck cancer patients.

HOSPICE:

Hospice Education Institute
Three Unity Square
P.O. Box 98
Machiasport, ME 04655
800-331-1620
www.hospiceworld.org

This organization helps patients and their families to locate support services in their communities.

National Association for Home Care
228 Seventh St., SE
Washington, DC 20003
202-547-7424
www.nahc.org
The NAHC provides educational materials and information to determine how to choose home care and hospice providers.

National Hospice and Pallative Care Organization
1700 Diagonal Road, Ste. 625
Alexandria, VA 22314
800-658-8898 (helpline) or 703-837-1500
www.caringinfo.org
Free resources, including advance directives via web, email, and a toll-free helpline.

KIDNEY CANCER:

Kidney Cancer Association
1234 Sherman Avenue, Ste. 203
Evanston, IL 60202
800-850-9132
www.kidneycancerassociation.org
The Kidney Cancer Association provides printed information about the diagnosis and treatment of kidney cancer. The organization is dedicated to increasing funding for research, getting new drugs tried and approved, and supporting patients.

LEUKEMIA & LYMPHOMA:

The Leukemia & Lymphoma Society
1311 Mamaroneck Ave., Ste. 310
White Plains, NY 10605
800-955-4572 or 914-949-0084
www.lls.org
This organization covers the main blood cancers: leukemia, lymphoma, and multiple myeloma. This organization provides information, support, medical news on a regular basis, and patient financial aid.

Lymphoma Research Foundation
115 Broadway, 13th Floor
New York, NY 10006
800-235-6848 or 212-349-2910
www.lymphoma.org
The LRF funds research and provides educational information on lymphoma. Lymphoma patients can receive free information customized to their diagnosis and find clinical trials and peer support information.

LUNG CANCER:

American Lung Association
61 Broadway, Sixth Floor
New York, NY 10006-2701
800-LUNGUSA (800-586-4872) or 212-315-8700
www.lungusa.org
This organization is dedicated to the prevention of lung disease and the promotion of lung health by focusing on environmental health, research and professional education, and advocacy, multicultural, and communications programs.

lungcancer.org
275 Seventh Ave.
New York, NY 10001
800-813-HOPE (800-813-4673) or 212-712-8400
www.lungcancer.org
This organization provides education, resources, clinical trial information, support groups, teleconferences, and an e-newsletter.

Lung Cancer Alliance
1747 Pennsylvania Ave. NW, Ste. 1150
Washington, DC 20006
800-298-2436 or 202-463-2080
www.lungcanceralliance.org
This is a nonprofit organization that advocates on behalf of lung cancer patients, survivors, families, caregivers, and those at risk. Its mission is to eliminate lung cancer. In addition it offers educational programs about lung cancer and provides support.

CANCER MAGAZINES:

Cancer & You Magazine
Griffin Publishing Group
P.O. Box 1605
Royal Oak, MI 48068
This magazine contains several articles on various aspects of cancer including treatment, drugs for cancer, notable patient interviews, and more. It is published by the McCarty Cancer Foundation in Royal Oak, Michigan as an information source for patients. It is distributed through pharmacies.

Caring4Cancer
P4 Healthcare LLC
6031 University Blvd. Ste. 235
Ellicott City, MD 21043
www.caring4cancer.com
This quarterly publication provides help to guide cancer survivors and caregivers with practical knowledge and inspiration.

Articles include a broad range of topics such as treatment, financial assistance, nutritional advice, complimentary medicine, caregiving, and moving forward.

Coping Magazine
P.O. Box 682268
Franklin, TN 37068
615-790-2400
www.copingmag.com
Covers many different aspects of survivorship, including psychological, emotional, and life after treatment.

Cure Magazine
3500 Maple Avenue, Ste. 750
Dallas, TX 75219
800-210-CURE (800-210-2873) or 214-367-3500
www.curetoday.com
Publishes quarterly and covers many aspects of cancer especially for the newly diagnosed, including updates, research, and education.

Heal Magazine
3500 Maple Avenue, Ste. 750
Dallas, TX 75219
800-210-CURE (800-210-2873) or 214-367-3500
www.healtoday.com
This magazine's emphasis is on survivorship post diagnosis and after initial treatment.

MULTIPLE MYELOMA:

International Myeloma Foundation
12650 Riverside Drive, Ste. 206
North Hollywood, CA 91607-3421
800-452-2873 or 818-487-7456
www.myeloma.org

IMF is dedicated to improving the quality of life of myeloma patients while working toward prevention and a cure. The organization provides information, research funding, seminars, and workshops for the blood disease multiple myeloma. IMF operates a Myeloma Hotline for the patient community and medical professionals.

McCarty Cancer Foundation
27172 Woodward Ave., Ste. 300
Royal Oak, MI 48067
800-746-0355 or 248-336-2500
www.cancerfoundation.org
The McCarty Foundation provides support for myeloma patients and funds research grants to fight myeloma on an annual basis.

Multiple Myeloma Research Foundation
383 Main Ave., Fifth Floor
Norwalk, CT 06851
203-229-0464
www.multiplemyeloma.org
MMRF provides educational materials and is very proactive in funding research for myeloma. This organization also sponsors patient/family seminars and teleconferences on multiple myeloma across the country. MMRF provides a bimonthly email newsletter with updates on research, a clinical studies database, and current topics on multiple myeloma. MMRF also sponsors an annual blood advocacy initiative in Washington, D.C.

OVARIAN CANCER:

Conversations: The International Overian Cancer Connection
P.O. Box 7948
Amarillo, TX 79114
806-355-2565
www.ovarian-news.org
This organization focuses on developing awareness and understanding of ovarian cancer. Publishes a free monthly

newsletter that provides hope, humor, support, and information about treatment and coping with ovarian cancer. Peer support is available.

National Ovarian Cancer Coalition (NOCC)
500 NE Spanish River Blvd., Ste. 8
Boca Raton, FL 33431
888-OVARIAN (888-682-7426) or 561-393-0005
www.ovarian.org
NOCC provides educational materials on ovarian cancer to promote awareness of the disease. They also provide a helpline, website, peer support, publications, and awareness projects.

Ovarian Cancer National Alliance (OCNA)
910 Seventeenth St., NW, Ste. 1190
Washington, D.C. 20006
202-331-1332
www.ovariancancer.org
OCNA provides advocacy for funding research for ovarian cancer. An annual advocacy conference is sponsored for survivors and families.

The Ovarian Cancer Research Fund (OCRF)
14 Pennsylvania Plaza, Ste. 1400
New York, NY 10122
800-873-9569 or 212-268-1002
www.ocrf.org
This organization focuses on funding research for early detection and development of new therapies. OCRF also promotes awareness of ovarian cancer with education programs, videos, and other resource information.

PAIN MANAGEMENT:

American Pain Foundation
888-615-PAIN (888-615-7246)
www.painfoundation.org
This organization provides a Pain Action Guide and offers
information, support, and advocacy.

PANCREATIC CANCER:

Pancreatic Cancer Action Network (PanCAN)
2141 Rosecrans Ave., Ste. 7000
El Segundo, CA 90245
877-272-6226 or 310-725-0025
www.pancan.org
This nonprofit advocacy organization provides educational
materials for the public and provides information on clinical
studies, support networks, and awareness.

PHARMACEUTICAL REIMBURSEMENT:

Amgen Reimbursement Connection
800-272-9376
www.amgen.com/patients/assistance.html

Bristol-Myers Squibb Patient Assistance Foundation
800-736-0003
www.bmspaf.org

CancerCare
800-813-HOPE (800-831-4673)
www.cancercare.org

Celegene Patient Support Solutions Program
(Assistance for Thalomid and Revlimid)
888-423-5436, option 3

Cephalon, Inc.
(Trisenox Reimbursement and Patient Assistance Hotline)
866-261-7730

Genentech Access Solutions
866-4-ACCESS (866-422-2377)
www.spoconline.com

GlaxoSmithKline's Commitment to Access
1-8-ONCOLOGY1 (866-265-6491)
www.commitmenttoaccess.gsk.com

Lilly Cares
800-545-6962
www.lillycares.com

Millennium Pharmaceuticals, Inc.
(VELCADE Reimbursement Assistance Program)
1-866-VELCADE (866-835-2233)

NeedyMeds
www.needymeds.com
The website provides a list of prescription assistance programs available from drug companies. Note that patients cannot apply directly to these programs. You need to have a doctor, nurse, or social worker contact NeedMeds on your behalf.

Novartis
(Reimbursement Hotline for Zometa)
866-4-ZOMETA (866-496-6382)

Ortho Biotech Inc.
(Reimbursement Hotline for Doxil)
800-609-1083

Partnership for Prescription Assistance
888-4PPA-NOW (888-477-2669)
www.pparx.org

Patient Advocate Foundation
866-512-3861
www.copay.org

Pfizer Helpful Answers
866-776-3700
www.pfizerhelpfulanswers.com

Rx Hope
877-979-4673 or 732-507-7400
www.rxhope.com

Sanofi-Aventis's PACT Plus
800-996-6626
oncology.sanofi-aventis.us

Schering-Plough's Commitment to Care Program
800-521-7157
www.schering-plough.com

Together Rx Access
800-444-4106
www.togetherrxaccess.com

PROSTATE CANCER:

American Foundation for Urologic Disease
1128 N. Charles St.
Baltimore, MD 21201
800-242-2383 or 410-468-1800
www.afud.org
This nonprofit organization's website includes information on prostate cancer for the public, as well as a support network for prostate cancer patients, families, and survivors.

Arnie's Army Battles Prostrate Cancer
20 Westport Rd.
Box 855
Wilton, CT 06897
866-586-5585
www.arniesarmybattles.com
This charity golf event is designed to raise prostate cancer awareness.

National Prostate Cancer Coalition
1154 Fifteenth St. NW
Washington, DC 20005
888-245-9455 or 202-463-9455
www.fightprostatecancer.org or www.4npcc.org
This prostate organization uses awareness, outreach, and advocacy to make life easier for men dealing with prostate cancer.

Prostate Cancer Foundation
1250 Fourth St.
Santa Monica, CA 90401
1-800-757-CURE (800-757-2873)
www.prostatecancerfoundation.org
This foundation is the world's largest philanthropic source of support for prostate cancer research.

Prostate Cancer Research Institute (PCRI)
5777 West Century Blvd., Ste. 800
Los Angeles, CA 90045
800-641-7274 or 310-743-2116
www.pcri.org
The objective of PCRI is to educate patients and their families about prostate cancer, including new advances in diagnosis, staging, treatments, and available resources.

US Too! International Inc.
5003 Fairview Ave.
Downers Grove, IL 60515
800-80-US TOO (800-808-7866) or 630-795-1002
www.ustoo.org
Us Too! is a support group for prostate cancer and includes educational information for newly diagnosed prostate cancer patients and the latest data on treatment. It has 325 chapters worldwide.

SARCOMA:

The Sarcoma Alliance
775 East Blithedale, #334,
Mill Valley, CA 94941
415-381-7236
www.sarcomaalliance.com
The Sarcoma Alliance provides education, support, help finding medical providers, treatment options, and other information sources.

Sarcoma Foundation of America
9884 Main St.
P.O. Box 458
Damascus, MD 20872
301-520-7648
www.curesarcoma.org
This organization raises funds for sarcoma research, patient networking, and support.

SKIN CANCER:

Melanoma International Foundation
250 Mapleflower Rd.
Glenmoore, PA 19343
888-463-6663 or 610-942-3432
www.melanomaintl.org
Educates the public on prevention and early detection of
melanoma, provides educational programs, and operates a toll-free
patient/family hotline.

The Skin Cancer Foundation
149 Madison Ave., Ste. 901
New York, NY 10016
800-SKIN-490 (800-754-6490)
www.skincancer.org
This foundation focuses on increasing awareness of skin cancer by
providing public and professional education, medical training, and
research.

SUPPORT ACTIVITIES:

CarePages, Inc.
4043 N. Ravenswood Ave., 301
Chicago, IL 60613
888-852-5521
www.carepages.com
The National Coalition for Cancer Survivorship sponsors this
website. It provides free, personal, private web pages that help
family and friends communicate when someone is facing illness.

Gilda's Club Worldwide
322 Eighth Avenue, Ste. 1402
New York, NY 10001
888-GILDA-4-U (888-445-3248)
www.gildasclub.org
This very proactive organization was founded in behalf of Gilda
Radner. It is an international network where men, women, and
children with cancer and their families and friends join together
to build social and emotional support as a supplement to medical
care in a free, nonresidential, home-like setting. People with all
kinds and stages of cancer are welcome in thirty locations in the
U.S. and Canada. Programs provided include, but are not limited
to, networking groups, wellness groups, potlucks, lectures, various
activities groups (art, yoga, color penciling, singing, etc.)—all with
learning, sharing and fun in mind.

Reel Recovery
160 Brookside Rd.
Needham, MA 02492
800-699-4490
www.reelrecovery.org
Reel Recovery is a national nonprofit organization that conducts
free fly-fishing retreats for men recovering from life-threatening
cancer.

Reeling and Healing
1400 North State Pkwy., #8A
Chicago, IL 60610
www.reelingandhealingmidwest.org
866-237-5725 or 616-855-4017
Reeling and Healing is a licensed charitable nonprofit comprised
entirely of volunteers who provide fly-fishing retreats for women
diagnosed with or surviving cancer.

Thyroid Cancer:

ThyCa: Thyroid Cancer Survivors' Association, Inc.
P.O. Box 1545
New York, NY 10159
877-588-7904
www.thyca.org
ThyCa provides free support services, education, outreach, awareness information, a newsletter, and a cookbook that can be downloaded. This organization also sponsors Thyroid Cancer Awareness Month and raises funds for thyroid cancer research. ThyCa holds workshops and an annual conference.

Transportation:

National Patient Travel Center
4620 Haygood Rd., Ste. 1
Virginia Beach, VA 23455
800-296-1217 (helpline) or 757-512-5287
www.patienttravel.org
This organization provides a national patient helpline for information about assistance for long-distance medical air transportation.

Air Charity Network
410 First Ave. NW
Rochester, MN 55901
877-621-7177
www.aircharitynetwork.org
Through its seven nonprofit organizations, it provides access to free air transportation to specialized medical facilities to those dealing with a crisis.

Corporate Angel Network
Westchester County Airport
One Loop Road
White Plains, NY 10604
866-328-1313
www.corpangelnetwork.org
Arranges free air transportation for cancer patients to/from cancer
centers.

YOUNG ADULTS:

Planet Cancer
314 E. Highland Mall Blvd., Ste. 306
Austin, Texas 78752
512-452-9010
www.planetcancer.org
Planet Cancer is an online community for young adults with
cancer that also offers retreats.

The Ulman Cancer Fund for Young Adults
PMB #505
4725 Dorsey Hall Drive, Ste. A
Ellicott City, MD 21042
888-393-FUND (888-393-3863) or 410-964-0202
www.ulmanfund.org
The Ulman Fund provides free support programs, education, and
resources to help young adults, their families, and friends coping
with cancer.

APPENDIX II
BOOK SUGGESTIONS

Armstrong, Lance and Sally Jenkins. *It's Not About the Bike, My Journey Back to Life*. New York: G.P. Putnam's Sons, 2000.

Armstrong, Lance and Sally Jenkins. *Every Second Counts*. New York: Broadway Books, 2003.

Buscaglia, Leo. *Love*. New York: Fawcett Crest Books, 1972.

Canfield, Jack, with Mark Victor Hansen, Patty Aubery, Nancy Mitchell, R.N., and Beverly Kirkhart. *Chicken Soup for the Surviving Soul, 101 Healing Stories About Those Who Have Survived Cancer*. Florida: Health Communications, Inc., 1996.

Chopra, Deepak. *The Seven Spiritual Laws of Success*. California: Amber-Allen Publishing and New World Library, 1994.

Cousins, Norman. *Anatomy of an Illness as Perceived by the Patient*. New York: W.W. Norton, 1979.

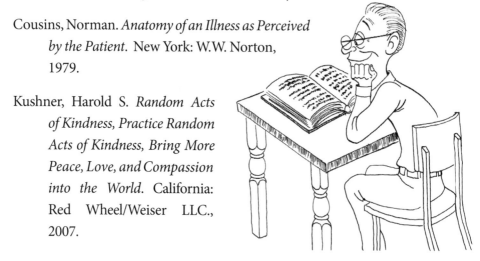

Kushner, Harold S. *Random Acts of Kindness, Practice Random Acts of Kindness, Bring More Peace, Love, and Compassion into the World*. California: Red Wheel/Weiser LLC., 2007.

Gibran, Kahlil. *The Prophet*. New York: Alfred A. Knopf, 1923.

Hay, Louise. *Everyday Positive Thinking*. California: Hay House, Inc., 2004.

Jacobs, Bert and John. *Life is Good. Simple Words from Jake and Rocket*. Iowa: Meredith Books, 2007.

Jordan, Hamilton. *No Such Thing As a Bad Day*. New York: Pocket Books, 2000.

Peale, Norman Vincent. *The Amazing Results of Positive Thinking*. New York: Fireside, 1959.

Peale, Norman Vincent. *The Power of Positive Thinking*. New York: Fireside, 1952.

Siegel, Dr. Bernie S. M.D. *How to Live Between Office Visits*. New York: HarperCollins, 1993.

Appendix III
Voices of Inspiration

In writing this book I came into contact with so many wonderful people with so many inspirational stories that I felt obligated to include some of them here. Each story generally covers three things: what that person's major life challenge was, what they did to turn around the adverse situa-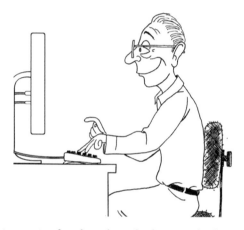tion, and what role (if any) positive attitude played in dealing with that challenge. My hope is that these stories can provide additional insight into how others have coped with adversity in their lives.

*   *   *   *   *

The major challenge of my life began with a diagnosis of multiple myeloma, a blood cancer that is considered incurable. For me, I think a positive attitude played a major role in dealing with the diagnosis, the difficult medical treatments, and my continual coping with the disease.

During these difficult times, I drew strength from my wife, who has always demonstrated a positive attitude since the day I was diagnosed with multiple myeloma. Together, we also used the power of prayer to guide, help, and comfort us. Our faith and trust in God was, and is, certainly a major factor in dealing with this adversity.

I also received inspiration and strength from my fellow members of the multiple myeloma support group at Gilda's Club. The courage and grit they showed in fighting this terrible disease were certainly the traits that I tried to emulate.

Larry Rushlow, four-year cancer survivor

*   *   *   *   *

My life has been one trauma after another, beginning when I was a small child. As I have gotten older, I have learned how important attitude is when trying to deal with trauma in a healthy way. Having an "attitude of gratitude" always helps.

The following actions help me cope with all my adversities:

Stay close to God and pray frequently. *Always maintain an attitude of gratitude.* No matter how bleak it looks, there is always something to be grateful for—keep your focus on that.

Spend as much time around animals as possible, preferably a dog. If you don't have a dog—borrow one for walks or volunteer at an animal shelter.

Express your feelings in a creative way. Paint, draw, sing, dance, write. Don't say you have no talent. Just do it. Act as if you have talent, and you might be surprised at what you can do.

Exercise daily—walk, walk, walk, breathe, breathe, breathe, pray, pray, pray.

Christine Emmick

*   *   *   *   *

The major challenge in my life is twofold: my being diagnosed with cancer (multiple myeloma) and my wife's diagnosis with dementia (Lewy Body Dementia).

The benefits of a positive attitude—as well as I could maintain it—were very instrumental in coping with our diseases. I can say very honestly that throughout these five-plus years of our diseases, I have never had a negative attitude. I'm not entirely sure why, but there are a number of factors that could explain it.

1. Praying. Specifically, during my six months of chemotherapy, I had frequent pains in the bowels, intestines, stomach, and more, and every time I would pray earnestly for relief, and every time God provided that relief.

2. As soon as I was diagnosed, there was a continuous flow of people caring for the two of us: cards, letters, phone calls, visits, meals brought to us, and rides taking us to many appointments. Their caring and their prayers were overwhelming. I have over two hundred cards, many with personal messages.

3. When I did get out of the house and met people I knew, so very many of them said how good I looked.

4. I am convinced that my being a caregiver for my wife for almost four years kept my focus away from my own disease. And the specific reason I chose to have a stem cell transplant was to maintain/improve my own health so I could take care of Carol as long as I could.

5. Support groups. For me, there were a few people who became good friends who also had multiple myeloma. But, I actually had even more experience with support groups through being the caregiver for Carol. There were Alzheimer's/Dementia support group meetings at our hospital, local health centers, assisted living and retirement communities, and local offices for associations dedicated to helping those affected by Alzheimer's.

6. I also did a lot of journaling. Even though I recall recording mostly factual things rather than my own feelings, and the notes I wrote are now scattered about in so many different places, it was definitely helpful for me in dealing with things.

7. Then there is Leanne, my infusion nurse at Providence Hospital. She was always there for me as my advocate—very encouraging. Plus, as she explained my plan of chemotherapy and shots of neuprogen, I was able to plot out the dates on the calendar, and I always could focus on exactly when the whole series would be over.

8. For exercise, I walked along the roadside picking up trash at least once a week.

9. I read about fifteen biographies or autobiographies that dealt with cancer and Alzheimer's.

In summary, early in my treatment I recall talking with so many people about my disease and my treatment—I found myself saying to them, "I'm going to beat this thing."

Edward Scharrer, five-year cancer survivor and caretaker for his wife with dementia

*　　*　　*　　*　　*

My major challenge was surviving the Holocaust. There were hundreds of scary, depressing, and tragic events, but what helped me endure and survive were my optimism, toughness, and courage—always believe in yourself and look toward tomorrow.

Mania Salinger, Holocaust survivor

*　　*　　*　　*　　*

I was hit by a drunk driver in November 1985. After six and a half months of intensive care and rehabilitation, I remained in a wheelchair, unable to walk, with what is called a T-6 injury. This was a result of a punctured aorta (lack of oxygen to the spinal cord), crushed rib cage, closed-head injury, spinal fusion, and multiple broken bones.

I went through the typical denial and anger stages, but the hatred was eating me up. I decided not to roll over and play dead, but to thank God for sparing my life. This positive outlook helped me to cope with my minute-to-minute challenges.

In order for me to get well emotionally, mentally, and physically, I initially listened and meditated to relaxation tapes (ocean waves, nature sounds, etc.). Then I did a lot of mental imaging (for example, my lungs became the Goodyear blimp and my heart muscle became Hulk Hogan). It also helped me to speak to church, school, and business groups about my accident—not only how I mourned the loss of my legs daily, but how I compensated with other activities. God has been good to me! He has given me the strength to raise two children, teach special education, remarry, and go on with a productive and healthy life!

Kathleen Haines Dailey, accident paralysis survivor

*　*　*　*　*

My three-year-old daughter had a very high fever and was very lethargic, so we took her to the hospital. There we learned that she was close to death with a (subsequently determined) blood infection. She had to lie on a bed of ice with essentially no clothes on and was in the hospital for several days.

In this case it was very important for her mother and me to present a positive attitude. Young children easily detect your emotions (and this was a very intelligent young lady for her age!). While our daughter could not quite understand what was happening to her, she was greeted consistently with our very positive demeanor and sincerity of conversation. This was important not only for our daughter, but for us as the parents as well.

Among the ways that we used to deal with this situation were to rationalize our way through the few things that seemed to be on our side. I discussed with my wife how strong-willed our daughter was, that she was smart enough to follow directions (from the doctor, nurse, us, etc.), and that because she was such a *thinker*, that we would converse with her in a way to make her think not only about what she had to do, but also about other subjects to get her mind off of her physical condition. Through identifying "what is right or good" and focusing on that appropriately, one can and will get through the crisis.

Michael Ricco, parent of seriously ill daughter

*   *   *   *   *

At forty-six, I was diagnosed with stage-two bilateral breast cancer. This meant chemotherapy, then radiation, followed by more chemotherapy. From start to finish (first mammogram to last chemo), it was fifteen months.

After doing some research and reading, I came to believe that attitude was as important as the chemo and radiation. I read a great deal of Bernie Siegel and *Anatomy of an Illness as Perceived by the Patient* by Norman Cousins, which convinced me that positive attitude and laughter could help.

I prayed for guidance and strength. I read Bernie Siegel and listened to his humor and visualization tapes. I re-read my collection of Louis L'Amour books (in which the good guy always wins) and other authors with whose writings had similar outcomes, and I avoided authors whose books did not reflect life with positive outcomes. I enjoyed movies like the *Lethal Weapon* series (incredibly violent, but also incredibly funny, and the good guy wins). I looked for the ridiculous in frustrating situations, and often was able to laugh at others getting pissed at things that were unimportant in the grand scheme of life. I tried to allow myself only to deal with people whose attitude mirrored mine and looked for occasions when we could laugh together.

Anonymous eleven-year breast cancer survivor

*　　　*　　　*　　　*　　　*

We really don't know when it started exactly. But we soon found out that it would change our lives forever. At the time I was raising three small boys. The "it" I talk about is the Alzheimer's my father had before his death, which was soon followed by the same disease my mother is still living with today. It all started over twenty years ago. My kids couldn't understand what was going on with Grandpa and Grandma—they couldn't remember the kids' names, or sometimes even that there were three children!

I was totally confused and frustrated, so I turned to my friends. Some of them knew of this disease and could explain. For me, it is day-by-day learning. I am learning patience, more for my Mom than my kids. I pray a lot and cry a lot. After I visit her, I often leave crying. But then I pull myself together because, after all, Mom is not in any pain. She is very happy and content. She is not in my world, but she is very happy in hers. I leave and try to treat myself to something nice.

I want my old Mom back. I miss my Dad. I have a very loving husband who is very supportive. We also had to deal with it in his Mom. My friends try to understand and are there for me when I need them. My birds, I thank God for my birds. God knows how much they have done to help me get through it.

I deal and I cope the best I can. And that's all we can do: *the best we can.* My Mom will be ninety-six in October of this year. I love her deeply and always will. I have come to terms with the fact that as long as she loves me it will be okay. She has become very fragile, very frail. Every moment is special.

For those of you going through the same thing or something similar, you have my prayers. Turn to faith, friends, animals, whatever it takes. See a therapist. Join a support group. I have started a family counseling group at the community where Mom lives. It is going strong! And I do have my support, and that's what gets me through it all.

Kathy Tromblay, dealing with parents with Alzheimer's

*   *   *   *   *

Most of the major challenges in my life have, interestedly enough, come recently in my life (I am forty years old). Over the last seven years, a major challenge has been to be a good parent to my daughter. I am helping raise her along with my ex-girlfriend. The major challenge is that my ex-girlfriend and I do not get along at all, and this severely limits how good we can be as parents to our daughter. Also, to complicate matters, my ex-girlfriend has bipolar mood disorder and has not been getting treatment for it. On top of that, about four months ago I was diagnosed with cancer. Finally, two months ago I was laid off from work and am now unemployed, with a potential financial crisis looming in the near future.

My positive attitude has been hugely beneficial in dealing with all of life's stresses. I have always tried to have a positive, "the cup is half full" attitude, and recent events have put this philosophy to the maximum test.

I have taken action in several ways to deal with my recent challenges. Going to Gilda's Club has been a huge help in dealing with cancer by talking with friendly people who are in similar situations to myself. It is a great community of compassionate people. I love it there, and I will continue to go for a long time. Also, I have been doing a lot of reading, and I have started studying Buddhism. I have gone to a couple of Buddhist services, and I also love their spirit and community. It is bringing me relief from suffering, it is liberating, and I enjoy it. I hope to learn more and take it up on a more permanent basis.

John Persons, cancer survivor and single parent

*   *   *   *   *

In 1967 (the year I turned nineteen), my father died of leukemia and my mother was diagnosed with breast cancer. She survived for another thirty-two years. In 2002, my own "nothing to worry about" bump was diagnosed as advanced and aggressive parotid cancer.

I had read Bernie Siegel, Norman Cousins, and Louise Hay, and I knew that visualization, laughing, and having a positive attitude and a sense of humor would help—and they certainly have.

To deal with everything and maintain my positive attitude, I watched TV and DVDs (*Shrek* particularly helped me in radiation burn) and read funny books. I also meditated and listened to Bernie Siegel tapes. In the hospital I watched the "New Age"/travel sites channel—the soothing music and the pretty vistas (beaches, waterfalls, etc.) helped to keep me relaxed.

Stuart G. Itzkowitz, five-year head and neck cancer survivor

*   *   *   *   *

I was diagnosed with breast cancer in January 2003.

I knew it was up to me to heal from this disease. After diagnosis, I was in shock for a few days. Then I said to myself, "You must decide—either you take control of this disease or the disease will take control of you." It was all up to me!

I knew my attitude would also play a big role in my healing. I had a choice every day—have a pity party for myself, or take control of the situation. If you have a positive attitude, things will come to you. You open yourself so that Spirit can send healing energy your way. The saying goes, "You must be open and receptive." I have found this to be so true. A negative attitude will bring more negativity to you; a positive attitude will bring the positive to you!

To maintain my positive attitude, I did a lot of reading, meditation, and loving myself. I attended classes on healing touch, EFT (emotional freedom technique), detoxification of my organs, and general health and nutrition. I sought out the help of others who had gone through the same thing. I also joined a breast cancer group at Gilda's Club and a group called Reeling and Healing Midwest, which offers fly-fishing retreat weekends for women undergoing breast cancer therapy. And I got involved with helping others.

I also took on daily positive affirmations, which I practice to this day. Every time I saw a mirror or reflection of myself I said, "You are in perfect radiant health!" I believe the body responds to thoughts and attitudes—by being positive, you bring about positive in your life.

I have a quotation on my desk entitled "Attitude," by Charles Swindoll; I thought I'd share it:

> The longer I live, the more I realize the impact of attitude on life.
>
> Attitude, to me, is more important than facts. It is more important than the past, than education, than money, than circumstances, than failures, than successes, than what other people think or say or do. It is more important than appearance, giftedness, or skill. It will make or break a company . . . a church . . . a home.
>
> The remarkable thing is we have a choice every day regarding the attitude we will embrace for that day. We cannot change our past. We cannot change the fact that people will act in a certain way. We cannot change the inevitable.
>
> The only thing we can do is play on the one string we have, and that is our attitude. I am convinced that life is 10 percent what happens to me, and 90 percent how I react to it. And so it is with you . . . we are in charge of our attitudes.

Finally, it was also important to me to be a role model for my two girls. By having a positive attitude, I believe I taught them the meaning of attitude in life. Bad things will always come up during your lifetime—you can't stop them. But you do have a choice in how you will deal with them—attitude means so much in the way you deal with adversity. What legacy do you want to leave? Having a positive attitude will live in hearts forever.

Carolyn Rushlow, four-year breast cancer survivor

*   *   *   *   *

My husband, Ken, and I had a plan to sell our nice home and purchase two other more modest homes: one for rental and one for restoration, ultimately to sell for a profit. The day after we closed on these properties, Ken was rushed to the hospital in horrible pain, becoming paralyzed before my eyes. He was diagnosed with Guillain-Barre syndrome (a nerve disorder).

The dream we had together was now turning into a nightmare, one that I might have to face alone. As my husband lingered in the hospital, bills were piling up at home. The feeling that everything we worked for was fast floating away caused me nearly overwhelming anxiety. And the question arising over and over was, "Why us?" And then I thought, of course us! God recognizes that we can handle this. He allowed us to raise and enjoy every day with our children, we never suffered financially, and we had a joyous marriage filled with love and happiness. Just realizing this made the challenges of this illness bearable. We would get through this together, whatever the outcome, because God loved us enough to call on us to find a way.

After many months, my husband did make a wonderful recovery; he was, however, unable to return to work. Our dreams of making a million dollars now seem unimportant; we did what needed to be done, adjusted our lives accordingly, and now can see joy in every day because we are together! Leaning on faith, I kept repeating, "God never gives you more than you can handle." This thought, and focusing on doing normal things every day, made the overwhelming bearable and gave me time to be *me*.

Patricia Gauvreau, spouse and caregiver for husband in his illness

*   *   *   *   *

I was hit with chronic fatigue syndrome and fibromyalgia about eighteen years ago. It caused me horrible pain, and fatigue that is far beyond what you can imagine unless you've had it yourself. It feels like your brain is filled with a dark cloud that doesn't go away. Along with this comes depression, weight gain, and an inability to think or work.

My faith in God, reading scripture when I was able to read, gave me something to hold onto and believe in. Sometimes I watched cartoons or funny movies to help. I'd listen to music to feel like I was still participating in life, and watching some Christian television. Praying to God and saying scripture out loud was the best help against depression.

Anonymous eighteen-year survivor of chronic fatigue syndrome and fibromyalgia

*   *   *   *   *

My life, like others, has gone through many challenges: death of loved ones, cancer of three family members, a brother near death with life-threatening meningitis, a car accident that left a family member paralyzed for life, and rescues from a near-drowning accident. Also, during my educational career, I was able to successfully intervene and confiscate drugs from a student who was holding other teachers at gunpoint. But the longest and most constant challenge of my life was the career path I chose, which was filled with both adversity and diversity of human conditions for over thirty years. I taught special education and worked with mentally, physically, and emotionally impaired children between the ages of eight and twenty-five years old.

A positive attitude, combined with the ability to perceive and understand both my needs as well as those of another, is vital to surviving major challenges. People need people! We are social animals with varying levels of wills that help us cope and live. A positive attitude is a reflection that helps others to believe in their own personal strengths and to direct their lives in a healthier direction. Like a battery, being positive re-energizes your soul and gives you the energy for life's challenges.

I like humor! It can change our thoughts so that we are not so focused on ourselves. Humor is the oil that lubricates us so that we can handle life's challenges. Having a good mindset heals our body and tends to enhance our soul. To cope with life's challenges, we must choose love, joy, and life versus loneliness, hate, and despair. I still find the Boy Scout Oath, Law, and Motto a good guide to facing everyday life. Having a conscience to care and to always let other people who are close to you know how much you care about them gives me the desired outcome of peace and love.

I also offer this quote from an unknown author: "The nature of gravity dictates that it is impossible for the bumblebee to fly. The nature of the bumblebee dictates that it will." The quote continues with an explanation: "People exceed their capabilities all the time when they're not aware that what they're doing is 'impossible.' If it were really human nature to believe something is impossible, no child would ever 'fly.'"

Larry Ricco, retired special education teacher

*   *   *   *   *

I had breast cancer and cancer in the lymph nodes, which was treated with one year of chemo and a very intense recovery. One of my coping techniques was humor; I watched comic videos, "I Love Lucy," "Cheers," and some tapes sent by my son. These made me laugh, and they let me begin to breathe again and talk about my cancer with others. Talking about it also allowed me to become a resource for many of my friends, and I began to take friends to doctor appointments and help others to cope with their own problems.

Betty Patullo, breast cancer survivor

*   *   *   *   *

My major challenge in life has been a severe hearing impairment. Sometimes, I hear people incorrectly or misunderstand. I often feel left out of some conversations. I try to tell people upfront that I have a hearing problem so that they look at me directly or speak louder. A sense of humor helps! But it doesn't solve everything. So to cope with the rest, I try to read a lot so I may keep growing. I also rent only movies with subtitles.

I offer this poem that I wrote:

Overcoming Adversity, When You Believe

The clock kept on ticking through
the night
I lay there thinking until the
morning light
How can I overcome this grim
prediction of fate?
"I love life and my family", and
while reflecting. I silently wait . . .

I remember my childhood, happy
and free
My perfect health and days filled
with glee
Plans for the future seemed to fit
into place
Now, in a mirror reflection, I see
my face!

The doctor seemed hopeful as I
sat in the chair
He smiled and kept talking, yet I

felt so unaware
I knew that for me to overcome my
fears and obstacles,
I would need a group gathering
where I
could relate and share

I went back in my mind to my
childhood faith
Trusting in His infinite mercy each
day
Lifting up my adversity and my
supplication
Asking God to just show me the
way!

As humans, we are so fragile and
weak
Our plans go amiss and lose their
power
I ask for His direction to bring me
through my mission in life
Until my final moment and hour!

"Don't give up on me Lord, I know
your
Plan must be complete
you are not finished with me yet
Let me not faint or give up in
defeat!"

"Breathe into me the fight of Your
holy angels

Yet give me gentleness and the
tender
grace to accept Your will
Warm my heart with a feeling of
true peace and love
Take away uncertainty and night's
futile chill!"

JoAnna Folland Mazure, severe hearing impairment

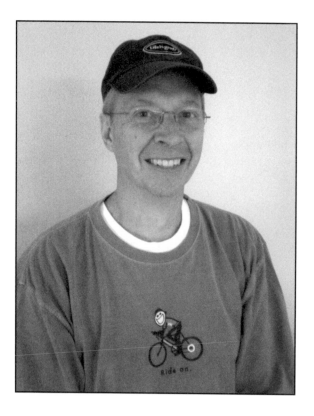

ABOUT THE AUTHOR

John Ricco is a seven-year cancer survivor, diagnosed at age fifty-two with multiple myeloma in June 2000. Retired from a more than thirty-year career in accounting and finance, he now devotes his time to helping others through active involvement in Gilda's Club, the Knights of Columbus, and other support and volunteer groups. He and his wife Jan reside in Farmington Hills, Michigan, where they have raised three wonderful daughters. *The Ride of Your Life* is his first book.